CAREGIVING
ACROSS CULTURES

CAREGIVING ACROSS CULTURES:
Working with Dementing Illness and Ethnically Diverse Populations

Ramón Valle, PhD

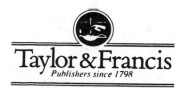

Taylor&Francis
Publishers since 1798

USA	Publishing Office:	Taylor & Francis 1101 Vermont Avenue, NW, Suite 200 Washington, DC 20005-3521 Tel: (202) 289-2174 Fax: (202) 289-3665
	Distribution Center:	Taylor & Francis 1900 Frost Road, Suite 101 Bristol, PA 19007-1598 Tel: (215) 785-5800 Fax: (215) 785-5515
UK		Taylor & Francis Ltd. 1 Gunpowder Square London EC4A 3DE Tel: 0171 583 0490 Fax: 0171 583 0581

CAREGIVING ACROSS CULTURES: Working with Dementing Illness and Ethnically Diverse Populations

1 2 3 4 5 6 7 8 9 0 E B E B 9 0 9 8 7

This book was set in Times Roman. The editors were Alison Labbate and Kathleen Savadel. Cover design by Joe Kolb.

A CIP catalog record for this book is available from the British Library.
∞ The paper in this publication meets the requirements of the ANSI Standard Z39.48-1984 (Permanence of Paper)

Library of Congress Cataloging-in-Publication Data

Valle, Ramón.
   Caregiving across cultures : working with dementing illness and ethnically diverse populations / Ramón Valle.
     p.   cm.
   Includes bibliographical references and index.

    1. Dementia—Patients—Care. 2. Transcultural medical care.
3. Minorities—Medical care. 4. Minorities—Services for. I. Cook
II. Title.
RC521.V34   1997
362.1'9683—dc21

                                                    97-30918
                                                     CIP

1-56032-529-1 (case: alk. paper)
1-56032-530-5 (ppk: alk paper)

To Jody Valle, my most dear and supportive wife.
To my children, Laura, Teresa, and Daniel,
and to Katalina Santibañez, my granddaughter.
May she grow up in an interculturally understanding world.

To Maria Victoria Valle, aunt and exemplary caregiver.

This work is dedicated to the many ethnically diverse dementia-affected elders
and their loving family members who were served over the years.
Their courage in the face of a most devastating disease
has provided the inspiration for this book.

Contents

PART TWO   INTEGRATION OF CULTURAL MAPPING CONCEPTS

List of Cases, Figures, and Boxes

CASES

FIGURES

BOXES

Preface

GOAL OF THE TEXT

This is a practice-oriented book. The text is a salute to those practitioners, at whatever level of dementia-care services, who are currently bringing much-needed assistance to dementia-impacted, ethnically diverse populations that are virtually cut off from existing mainstream diagnostic and treatment services. Enough cannot be said of these individuals throughout the country who are daily extending themselves in culturally relevant ways. It is hoped that this group of intercultural practitioners will find confirmation of their own competencies within the pages of this text.

This book is written with two primary audiences in mind. First, it is directed to those interculturally experienced professionals and providers whose competencies have been honed by long years of experience with linguistically and culturally diverse clients seeking relief from the wrenching effects of dementing illness striking a loved one at the heart of the family. The second intended audience consists of those professionals or providers who are beginners within the intercultural arena. It may be that the interest has just been sparked, or that some initial steps have already been undertaken. However, in both instances the practitioner is looking for direction.

There is also a possible third audience, namely researchers and their parent investigative organizations who are likewise seeking to engage ethnoculturally diverse groups. Although culturally relevant research approaches will not be specifically highlighted, investigators will find that many of the cultural engagement working principles elucidated throughout the text can be adapted to many types of field studies and/or clinical trials targeting specific ethnic populations.

The intent of the text is to provide a working guide for the acquisition and/or refinement of intercultural engagement skills through the application of what are termed *cultural mapping techniques* for all of the groups. As defined here, *cultural mapping* can be described as a multifaceted assessment strategy that centers on identifying the core linguistic–communicational patterns, customs, and coping strategies, as well as the value frameworks of the ethnically diverse groups and their affiliated members. Cultural mapping makes use of what is outlined below as the *acculturation continuum model*. This framework assists the practitioner in sorting traditional, culture-of-origin perspectives, bicultural outlooks, and acculturated-to-the-host-society views in relation to the ethnically diverse populations targeted for dementia-care assessments and interventions.

The text will deal with many facets of intercultural practice within the overarching cultural mapping concept. *Part One: The Cultural Mapping Process in Dementia Services* centers around the professional or provider, beginner or experienced, seeking to contact and interact with an ethnically diverse clientele. It is directed toward the direct-service staff member in the organization, or in the field, along with the service manager and the organization from which the contacts or services originate. The emphasis throughout Part One is on highlighting skills that will help busy practitioners establish *intercultural rapport* within the scope of their cross-ethnic assignments. The discussion ranges from the presentation of techniques for understanding the roles to be performed and the skills inherent to making culturally appropriate assessments, through the practitioners acquiring the capability to distinguish between what is, and what is not culture. The discussion in Part One also spotlights important techniques for linking to the ethnic group members' traditions, values, and beliefs, as well as their cultural expectations around help-seeking and help-accepting practices.

A central tenet of the narrative in Part One is that the professionals' or the practitioners' attention has to be focused on maintaining dementia-affected elders and the ethnic family members' *cultural dignity*. In cross-cultural work it is not enough to be alert to the dignity of the individual. The professional or provider extending dementia-focused assistance to culturally diverse families must be equally attentive to preserving the dignity of the ethnocultural group-as-a-whole including the family's beliefs and customs and not just the dignity of the dementia-affected elder alone. Practitioners experienced in working with ethnically diverse families will easily recognize that the intercultural engagement process begins and ends with a focus on the collective coping abilities of family members and significant others involved in the situation of the dementia-affected elder (Gaines, 1988–1989, pp. 36–37).

Even when the family is conflicted, or where there may be no family directly involved, the memories of the person's collective extended family experience are a powerful dynamic among more traditionally oriented ethnic groups. It is important to keep in mind that this core element of human interaction can be extended to all ethnic groups, including people of Euro-ethnic heritage, who likewise hold to their traditional culture-of-origin orientations, be these related to a region of the country or to an era of the nation's history. The practitioner's efforts, therefore, cannot stay focused on what the literature terms *the primary caregiver alone*. It makes no difference how extended the caregiving group may be. From an intercultural engagement standpoint, the practitioner needs to assume that all are somehow involved. Beginners, to whom this important intercultural engagement principle might be new, must log it into their list of practice "must-do's." Moreover, the principle must be applied throughout the total process of engaging culturally and linguistically diverse clients.

Part Two: Integration of Cultural Mapping Concepts provides a brief intermediate summary of the intercultural mapping concepts outlined in Part One. It can serve both as a shortened overview and an encapsulation of the key principles involved in the intercultural engagement process.

Part Three: Supporting Intercultural Competency Development shifts the discussion to another level. The estimate, as of this writing, is that the bulk of effective dementia-oriented assessment and intervention activity is occurring at the level of the direct, "hands-on" staff. The multicultural reality of the social environment has not yet penetrated the management and service decision-making core of most dementia-focused organizations. This circumstance is often very disheartening to the professionals or providers struggling day in and day out, almost alone, trying to extend dementia services to culturally diverse consumers. They may be working very effectively with different ethnic group members, assisting these significant others caring for a dementia-affected elder. However, when these practitioners bring the patient and the family to the home agency, the reception can be less than culturally cordial. Their peers and superiors at the management level simply may not fully grasp the issues involved in developing culturally attractive and serviceable organizational settings in which the ethnically diverse client group is received with culturally attuned understanding.

Part Three outlines the manner in which the organization's staff and managers can collaborate to create a culturally attuned, multicultural engagement capability. Strategies are highlighted for bringing the governing board, administration, and staff together through mission redefinement, internal resource reallocation, and ongoing intercultural competency training. Additional intercultural strategies, such as interagency networking (Hardcastle, Wencour, & Powers, 1997) and linking to cultural brokers who can connect the organization and its staff to the ethnic communities being targeted for intercultural dementia service (Aranda, 1990; Valle, 1988–1989) are likewise featured. The overall strategy of agency competency development extends to include a presentation of message transculturation techniques. Here the organization as well as professionals and providers can design culturally relevant information about dementing conditions for dissemination to ethnically diverse populations (Anrow Sciences of Mandex, Inc., 1987; Cunningham, 1991–1992).

DEMENTIA AND INTERCULTURAL ENGAGEMENT

The issue at hand is that dementing illness does not respect cultural boundaries (Advisory Panel on Alzheimer's Disease, 1993; Baker, 1988; Heyman et al., 1991; Homma, Ishii, & Niina, 1994; Manubens et al., 1995; Pi, Olive, Roca, & Masana, 1996; Schoenberg, Anderson, & Haerer, 1985; Serby, Chou, & Franssen, 1987; Smyth, Whitehouse, Rust, & Khaana, 1988–1989; Valle, 1981). However, persons from different ethnic groups may respond in culturally distinct ways (Valle 1990a, 1994). Therefore, there is an urgency to extend dementia-related services for culturally diverse groups. Something must be done at the systems level to meet the emergent need. The task cannot be left solely to the direct-service practitioner and/or people with lower decision-making status within the organization. It is essential that the field of dementia care as a whole face up to its responsibilities in the intercultural engagement arena.

Ideally, dementia-focused organizations would opt *en masse* to become ethnically relevant. Realistically, however, it is recognized that there may be deep-seated resistances to accommodating culture within the fabric of dementia-care organizations providing diagnostic and treatment interventions. The likelihood, therefore, is that widespread movement in this direction will be slow for some period to come. Resources remain scarce, and admittedly the efforts to develop organizationwide intercultural capabilities would compete for these limited resources. For example, line staff, managers, and governing boards would require intercultural competency training. New staff with bilingual/bicultural skills relative to the specific ethnic groups being targeted for services would need to be located and hired throughout all echelons of the organization, not just at the "hands-on" level. Organizational objectives would have to be recast to make them congruent with a newly accepted intercultural mission.

Therefore, although the text is ostensibly aimed at the current dementia-care organization as a whole, it is really written for the new generation of managers who will come from the ranks of the present interculturally competent, dementia-capable professionals and providers, as well as the beginners who join in now to accept the challenge of adding cultural expertise to their practitioner repertoire.

A NOTE ON ILLUSTRATIVE CASES USED IN THE TEXT

A number of cases are used for illustrative purposes throughout the text. These cases come from the author's direct practice experience, as well as from those intercultural dementia-care experiences shared over the years by colleagues, especially those named in the Acknowledgments. All names, as well as places and times in which the events described took place, have been changed to protect the confidentiality of the persons originally involved. Any resemblance noted to actual persons or circumstances known to the reader are purely coincidental.

Acknowledgments

Acknowledgments are extended to Maria Aranda, PhD; Katie Maslow, MSW; Elaina Weiss, MSW; Jacobo Mintzer, MD; and Andre Armstrong, MPA, model dementia care practitioners in their respective fields, for their thoughtful and helpful guidance throughout the preparation of the book.

The Cultural Mapping Process in Dementia Services

Part One spotlights the key elements of the cultural mapping process that are needed by the professional and provider seeking to become culturally competent in the provision of dementia-related services to ethnically diverse populations. *Cultural mapping* is an assessment technique that enables the practitioner to identify the key cultural characteristics of an ethnic group being targeted for services.

Chapter 1 highlights the key issues surrounding the growing diversification of U.S. society.

Chapter 2 discusses the necessary first step for developing a sound cross-cultural interventive capability, namely, the need for practitioners to be well grounded within a conceptual framework through which to understand culture and cultural processes. Before engaging in intercultural work, the practitioner must have a framework within which to be able to map the role of culture in the everyday life experience of different ethnic populations. The chapter details the basic ingredients for acquiring cultural competency. It presents a specific cultural assessment tool, the *acculturation continuum formulation,* for this purpose. This acculturation model helps the practitioner to respond to the cultural variations that will be encountered when working with ethno-cultural groups within a host society such as the United States. The chapter also discusses a number of factors that can distort the cultural assessment process. These include sorting out the ethnic client group's socioeconomic and educational status, along with being able to account for the residual effects of discrimination and prejudice. All of these elements need to be clearly separated from cultural understandings if a cross-cultural assessment or intervention is to be undertaken.

Chapter 3 examines the next step in the cultural mapping process. It offers an overview of how the professional or provider can begin to document the target ethnic group's cultural–historical presence within the service region. The discussion covers both multicultural as well as culture-specific information-gathering approaches and techniques. The chapter notes that, although there is usually readily acquirable information about the different ethnic populations residing throughout the United States, the information about these same ethnic groups related to dementing illness may at times be quite limited and uneven. Suggestions are offered as to how professionals or providers can go about filling in the information gaps they encounter. Finally, the chapter addresses the need to avoid creating stereotypes. Emphasis must be placed on keeping ethnic group information-gathering processes constantly open to new information and to incorporating how the target ethnic group members are actually expressing their ethnicity in the context of the client–practitioner relationship.

Chapter 4 further refines the cultural mapping process, focusing on the ways in which practitioners can gain an understanding of the many different aspects of the language and communication processes of ethnic diverse groups being targeted for dementia-related services. Language and overall communication patterns provide key cultural points of entry for the professional or provider seeking to establish intercultural ties with ethnically diverse client group members.

Chapter 5 centers on assisting the practitioner to understand and access a target ethnic group's interactional patterns. Ethnocultural ingroup relational patterns serve as further vital indicators of the ethnic group members' cultural orientations. The chapter focuses on gaining an awareness of the cultural expectations in regard to establishing rapport and trust. It presents the view that, in many, if not most ethnic group dementia-related caregiving situations, the professional or practitioner will encounter a decision-influencing network rather than a single caregiver acting alone. Therefore, practitioners entering the intercultural arena must be prepared to work with more persons than just the primary caregiver alone. The care network may include a range of significant others who become a part of the overall caregiving situation. The chapter closes with the presentation of a range of techniques that can be used to identify the target ethnic group's interactive patterns.

Chapter 6 focuses on another basic cultural mapping ingredient, namely, acknowledging and engaging the target ethnic group's values, beliefs, and normative expectations. These values and expectations become particularly crucial to understanding the ethnic group members' help-seeking and help-accepting orientations and actions. The chapter discusses learning how to observe and identify the client group's values and beliefs and examines how such factors as cultural shame and the desire for privacy within the more traditional ethnic group extended family/significant other network can influence the assessment of needs and the actual design of the careplan. The chapter ends with a description of cultural mapping techniques for overcoming various types of value differences, problems, and misunderstandings.

Chapter 7 elaborates a number of considerations presented in Chapter 2 that serve to distort the "cultural" side of the cultural mapping process. The chapter deals with the fact that socioeconomic status, the residual effects of past or present discrimination, the circumstance of low social status, and not being literate can all become inappropriately entangled with cultural characteristics being identified within the cultural mapping assessment. Practitioners need to learn how to separate these factors from cultural elements in any assessment being conducted, especially because social status factors do not define the group's ethnicity. At the same time, social status factors are not to be ignored. They do have a role in explaining the position of many ethnically diverse groups within the society. Moreover, these considerations can come into play anywhere with the dementia-care assessment process. However, mixing social status concerns with ethnocultural variables not only can undermine the sensitivity and specificity of cultural mapping assessments being made but also can lead to the stereotyping of ethnically diverse groups as all coming from lower socioeconomic and social status positions. For these reasons, practitioners conducting the cultural mapping effort must be continuously aware of what exactly is being observed and where the information being gathered appropriately belongs.

The overall intent of Part One is to provide a detailed insight into the different aspects of the intercultural engagement/cultural mapping process. Part One further seeks to delineate the manner in which the practitioner can apply the acculturation continuum framework within the context of everyday interaction with ethnically diverse client populations.

Introduction to Issues
and Working Assumptions

In approaching the discussion of dementing illness among ethnically diverse populations and the development of appropriate interventive care strategies, a variety of questions need to be addressed. For instance, is late-onset dementing illness making its impact felt among ethnically diverse populations and their caregiving significant others? Where dementia is present, what are the caregiving dynamics among ethnically diverse populations that need to be defined and understood? How is the professional or provider to appropriately identify cultural concerns within the vast array of caretaking issues that accompany dementing illness? How is the practitioner to extend services to the full range of ethnically and linguistically diverse populations found in most service catchment areas? It is the intent of the text to respond to these questions as well as to many other concerns. However, before proceeding, the reader should be alert to the basic concepts and assumptions that guide the overall discussion.

THE NATURE OF DEMENTING ILLNESS

The terms *dementia* or *dementing illness* will see frequent use throughout this text. They are used to denote a range of conditions that manifest themselves among elderly people late in the life course of an individual, conventionally accepted as appearing at age 65+. Dementing conditions can be identified in terms of a cluster of symptoms that affect the elder's ability to carry out regular functions of daily living and that bring about dramatic changes in the relationships of the elder and immediate significant others. The symptom complex includes: (a) impairment of short-term memory functions that affect work or home-making task performance; (b) difficulties in performing familiar tasks; (c) problems with language; (d) disorientation as to time and place; (e) poor or decreased judgment; (f) problems with abstract thinking; (g) misplacing things, and also even being unaware of their misplacement; (h) changes in mood or behavior; (i) changes in personality; and (j) loss of initiative (Alzheimer's Association, 1995). What complicates the dementing illness picture is that, as reported more than a decade ago, there are more than 70 conditions incorporated under the category of *late life dementia* (U.S. Congress Office of Technology Assessment, 1987).

In the early stages of dementing illness the symptoms are often subtle and insidiously intrude themselves into many different aspects of the affected person's daily life as well as the lives of the elder's significant others. In the early stages, the symptoms are manifested neither altogether, at any one time, nor in a uniform manner.

In addition, dementing illness presents itself in many unique patterns (Liu, Lin, et al., 1991; Liu, Tsou, et al., 1991; Patterson & Bolger, 1994). For example, the symptomatology can occur progressively and sequentially, or the symptoms can present themselves in seemingly idiosyncratic ways in any given individual case (Lawton, 1994; Teri & Gallagher-Thompson, 1991). Another feature of dementing conditions is that the individual generally experiences a gradual but progressive diminution of cognitive and other faculties over time. Exceptions could include multi-infarct dementia, in which a sudden vascular accident can mark the beginning of an equally precipitous impairment of cognitive functioning. Estimates of the prevalence of dementing illnesses among U.S. mainstream elderly cohorts vary, ranging from 6%–10%.

The most common form of late-life dementing illness is Alzheimer's disease, which accounts for approximately 60% of all dementing illness among the elderly and is found in combination with about another 20% of related conditions. Unfortunately, as of this writing, the causes of Alzheimer's disease remain unknown, and there is still no available cure. There is much ongoing research activity in these areas.

WORKING ASSUMPTIONS

Collectively, the issues just delineated are of considerable importance for the professional or provider working in the area of dementing illness, especially for the practitioner seeking to engage ethnically diverse populations. However, basic dementia research and treatment questions will not be engaged within the body of the text that follows. Rather, the text will remain focused on the cultural impact of dementing illness. In this context, the discussion will proceed from the standpoint of a number of assumptions. It is important, therefore, that the practitioner be aware of the premises that guide the discussion, as there will be little subsequent discussion of them beyond their being outlined here.

Changed Social Environment

ASSUMPTION #1: The United States' social environment is undergoing rapid changes in its ethnic composition, and the dementia-care community needs to be alert to these changes.

What has quickly, although not always so quietly, happened over the last quarter century in the United States are the dramatic changes that have taken place in the nation's ethnic composition. The United States has always been a diverse country. However, the current rapid growth in its immigration and birthrate-based ethnically diverse population reflects broader, and more world-wide, population profile (Banks, 1995; Fine, 1995; McLemore, 1994; Sirkin, 1994; Sokolovsky, 1990, pp. 197–200). For example, demographic projections, using the 1990 census as the baseline, esti-mate that the Euro-ethnic heritage composition of the U.S. population will drop to 53% of the population, from its present 73%, by the year 2050 (Day, 1995). The gains to be made will be from ethnic group populations with heritages other than Europe. States such as California already have this population configuration (Morganthau, 1997). Moreover, this trend is already visible in many current service environments in which the professional or provider can find large segments of new elderly immigrants from different sectors of Africa, Latin America, and the Arabic countries of the Mid-east, as well as from India, Pakistan, Russia, and other eastern European nations. An accompanying trend is the accelerated growth of elderly people in the U.S. population (Day, 1995), along with the increase of ethnically diverse elderly, who in the past were often referred to as *minority elderly* (Day, 1995; Gibson, 1989; Manuel, 1982; Stanford & Torres-Gil, 1991; Valle, 1988–1989). Specifically, four generic ethnic elderly populations: African Americans, American Indians/Native Americans, Asian Americans, and Latinos/Hispanics have doubled in size in each of the last three cen-sus periods, beginning with 1970. In addition, there is a growing diversity within the different ethnic group cohorts themselves. For example, there are large numbers of newly arrived Latin American elderly from countries other than Mexico. The elderly of Caribbean cultural origin who are not Spanish speaking, such as Haitians (French/ Patois speaking) and Jamaicans (English speaking) have similarly begun to swell the ranks of the U.S. ethnically diverse aged population. The assumption to be made, therefore, is that whether dementia-care practitioners and their parent organizations are aware of it or not, their service environments have diversified.

Diverse Groups Are Affected by Dementia

ASSUMPTION #2: Ethnically diverse groups are affected by dementing illness, and the community dementia-care practitioner must be alert and respond to this reality.

Regrettably, dementing illness, as one manifestation of neurodegenerative dis-ease, appears not only to be present within ethnically diverse populations but is also on the rise. This trend is projected to continue for several decades—well into the next century (Lilienfeld & Perl, 1994). Dementia among ethnically diverse elderly people, as well as caregiver concerns, have been regularly reported in the literature for a number of years and have included both clinical and community-based populations (Advisory Panel on Alzheimer's Disease, 1993; Cox & Monk, 1990, 1993; Dungee-Anderson & Beckett, 1992; Henderson, 1992, 1996; Henderson & Gutierrez-Mayka, 1992; Henderson, Gutierrez-Mayka, Garcia, & Boyd, 1993; Hinrichen & Ramirez, 1992; Lawton, Rajagopal, Brody, & Kleban, 1992; Lockery, 1987, 1991; Mintzer, Loewenstein, Millor, Flores, & Rainerman, 1992; Mintzer & Macera, 1992; Morycz, Malloy, Bozich, & Martz, 1987; Mui, 1992; Mui & Burnette, 1994; Segal & Wykle,

1988–1989; Sotomayor & Curriel, 1988; U.S. Congress Office of Technology Assessment, 1990; Valle et al., 1989; Wood & Parham, 1990; Wykle & Segal, 1991; Yeo, Gallagher-Thompson, & Lieberman, 1996; Young & Kahana, 1995).

The trend of an increase in the total numbers of ethnically diverse elderly, coupled with the fact that there is, as yet, no cure for dementing conditions such as Alzheimer's disease, has considerable dementia-care implications (Larson & Imai, 1996). From a clinical perspective, the incidence of dementing illness among ethnically diverse populations will most likely go up. The reasoning is not that the *rates* of dementing illness will increase among ethnically diverse groups but rather that there will greater numbers of ethnically diverse elderly afflicted with dementing illness. For example, the prevalence of dementing illness could be said to be 6%–10% of a given population. The fact that the group will be larger in the future does not increase the percentage of affected people but rather their number, and so more and more dementia-care practitioners, and their parent organizations, will in turn be faced with the increased need to be able to work across cultural and linguistic frontiers.

Furthermore, it is interesting to find that some of the literature is beginning to suggest there may be different prevalence rates of dementia, as well as of the different kinds of dementia, for some ethnically diverse populations worldwide (Evans, 1992; Haddock & Santos, 1992; Hendrie et al., 1993, 1995; Heyman et al., 1991; Hovaguimian et al., 1989; Kramer, 1996; Lavine et al., 1991; Ogunniyi & Osuntokun, 1991; Osuntokun, Ogunniyi, Lekwauwa, Norton, & Pillay, 1992; Zhang, Anderson, Lavine, & Mantel, 1990). However, the core issue for the dementia-care practitioner in the U.S. cultural environment is that dementia-affected Latinos/Hispanics, Asian Americans, Native Americans/American Indians, and African Americans, along with other ethnically diverse elderly, will all be losing their memory, their reasoning capacities, and their control over motor functions, following the progressive degenerative course of dementing conditions as discussed above. This signifies that they, and their caregiving social network members, will be expressing themselves in very different languages and will hold different cultural belief system formats. It is the intent of the text to provide the culture-appropriate tools for the practitioner to meet the needs of the changing multicultural environment.

The Practitioner Must Be Dementia Capable

ASSUMPTION #3: The professional or practitioner must be dementia capable, that is, have symptom recognition, diagnostic, and dementing illness knowledge and be familiar with the supportive service systems.

The practitioner will find very little actual discussion of dementing conditions themselves throughout the text beyond what is needed to elaborate the issues being presented. If more information on dementia is needed, the reader is advised to turn to the many available published materials throughout the field of dementia care that treat dementing illness in depth. Therefore, for the purposes of this text it is assumed that professionals and providers working in the dementia-caregiving arena will either be well versed in their understanding of Alzheimer's disease and other dementing disorders or know where to go to obtain the necessary information. The professional or provider's knowledge base is also assumed to include an understanding of the symptom patterns (only briefly enumerated above) that are manifested at both the onset and in later phases of dementing conditions. It is likewise assumed that the practitioners will be equally knowledgeable about the procedures necessary to conduct a differential diagnosis of a specific dementing condition. Despite the identification of some possible genetic linkages to the risk of such disorders as Alzheimer's disease reported earlier in the decade (Saunders et al., 1993), the actual final diagnosis can still be made only after medically excluding the possibility of all other potential causes of the symptoms observed within the clinical evaluation. As indicated above, there are as many as 70 possible conditions that can produce dementia symptomatology, which include some factors such as medications, alcohol abuse, uncontrolled diabetes, severe Vitamin B-12 deficiency, along with a number of mental health–related conditions such as depression and other emotional states (U.S. Congress Office of Technology Assessment, 1987). All of these conditions can mimic the symptoms of dementing illness, particularly the early stages of the illness. Moreover, even then, the diagnosis is that of possible or probable Alzheimer's disease. A confirmed diagnosis can still be given only after an autopsy findings report.

Finally, the expectation is that the practitioner also will be knowledgeable about dementia-care services. The course of the dementing conditions, which may extend anywhere over one to two decades, can be expected to bring demands for multiple types of services. The expectation is that the practitioner, in an effort to obtain a foundation of assessment capabilities on which to build principles for intercultural engagement, will become better informed about dementing illness and the services that are available. The focus of the discussion will remain on developing understandings to address the cultural responses of the elders and their caregiving family members/significant others about the onset of dementing illness and the manner in which a cultural connection between need and services can be established.

Illness and Response Require Separation

ASSUMPTION #4: In working with ethnoculturally diverse populations, the practitioner must be able to separate the illness state brought about by a dementing condition and the ethnic group members' responses to the illness.

There is some emerging evidence of varying ways in which dementing conditions might be viewed by different ethnic groups. For example, Ross et al. (1997), in their Hawaii-based study, report the phenomenon of *silent dementia*. They documented the fact that the Japanese ethnic group members tended not to identify and/or report the early signs of a possible dementing illness. Rather, the ethnic group members tended to identify the symptoms of the dementing illness when the condition had progressed to its more severe phases. Such information, if further verified with other ethnocultural groups, has considerable clinical implications for the manner in which the ethnic group member copes in the earlier symptom stages.

Kleinman (1977, 1980, 1986a, 1986b) has long suggested that professionals or providers working with ethnically diverse groups separate the actual illness and the group members' coping responses. A specific condition may physiologically manifest itself similarly across cultures, but each cultural group may respond differently. Others have echoed this perspective with respect to dementing illness (Elliot, Di Minno, Lam, & Mei Tu, 1996; Henderson, 1996; Valle, 1990a). The text, therefore, focuses on the area of the illness response patterns of ethnoculturally diverse groups rather than the disease entity itself. In this manner, the practitioner seeking to initiate the intercultural engagement process will be able to tap not only into the ethnic group's individual family's/significant others' concept of what is taking place but also into the unique coping responses of the ethnic group,

CULTURE AND ETHNICITY: WORKING DEFINITIONS

Extensive use will be made of the concepts of *culture* and *ethnicity* throughout the discussion that follows. The reader needs to be aware that the literature provides multiple definitions of both, especially of culture (Agar, 1994; Herskovits, 1973; Samovar & Porter, 1995). Moreover, the two terms are at times used in a manner so close in meaning as to be almost interchangeable. The text will not attempt to resolve all of the underlying definitional issues. Instead, a more practical approach will be taken. First, the concept of *culture* will be used to encompass the sum total of the values and beliefs of a group. Culture also includes the group's commonly used customs, its linguistic–symbolic communication systems, and the artifacts that are produced and/or used by the members of a group (Agar, 1994; Brislin, 1993; Kluckhohn, 1965; Samovar & Porter, 1995). *Ethnicity* brings the added connotation of belonging to a specific cultural group with its unique language, customs, and attendant beliefs. In essence, ethnicity is the active expression of culture.

In practice, the concepts of ethnicity and culture are often intermixed, and the terms are used almost synonymously. Ethnicity has a more "interactional" or "group membership" flavor, whereas the notion of culture leans more in the direction of identifying the group's underlying linguistic–communicational and value–symbol systems. At times throughout this text the two terms may even be combined, as in the phrase *ethnocultural group*. Similarly, the terms *cross-cultural, cross-ethnic,* or *intercultural engagement* also will be used. The connotation implicit in all of these terms is that the professionals or providers are bridging from their own cultural orientations and practices to an individual or population group with diverse and different cultural orientations and practices.

The term *cross-cultural* sees widespread use in many fields and encompasses clinical interventions through research activity involving ethnically diverse groups. Similarly, the phrase *cross-ethnic* is seeing increased application in the service and research worlds. The construct of *intercultural engagement* is encountered more frequently in the clinical and/or community intervention context. Throughout the practitioner's or provider's extended contact with any specific ethnic group, the important consideration in the application of culture, ethnicity, and intercultural engagement is that every caregiving situation is filled with cultural considerations expressed through the individual's and the family's/significant others' ethnic group attitudes and behavior.

The Notion of Culture: Additional Refinements

With these commonalities noted, it is still important to examine the notion of culture more closely. Gudykunst (1994) talks broadly about culture as including anything that is human made. Kluckhohn (1965) gives the idea of culture a more "activist" role. He indicates that culture helps to both shape what we are as human groups and broader societies as well as to influence our future actions. Basically, culture permeates the fabric of human interactions at every level—past, present, and future. As Silva-Netto (1994) notes, culture provides a cognitive and emotional map to which people refer as they go through life. Cultural considerations play a definite role in how the caregiver and the family/significant others perceive the professional or provider. Cultural considerations influence the extent to which the professional's or the provider's advice and help will be accepted and followed. Therefore, if practitioners are not culturally competent in their overall cultural assessments, or in their interactions with ethnically diverse group members, there will most likely be a negative influence on the outcome of a planned assessment or intervention. As discussed in the text, culture cannot just be dismissed as a passive influence on the client–practitioner engagement situation; it is seen as playing a very active role in the interaction between the practitioner and the ethnically diverse client.

Ethnicity: A Further Clarification

The concept of ethnicity also bears a closer review. Ethnicity is defined as *membership in a specific social group* (Gudykunst, 1994), or one's social heritage (McLemore, 1994), based on three expressed cultural characteristics. First, the group members share, or have loyalty to, a common language. This shared language is usually different than English, but it could also be some variation of what is considered standard English. For example Appalachian Americans, who are descendants of Scottish–Irish immigration early in U.S. history (McLemore, 1994), can be seen as a distinct ethnic subgroup within the broader U.S. mainstream society (Flan, 1991). Professionals and providers must be able to understand and communicate within this different form of English (Harper & Lanz, 1996), especially interpreting the meaning of what is said relative to dementing illness and its accompanying symptoms.

> Case 1.1. The practitioner working in an Appalachian community in eastern Tennessee was getting information about a mother's mood-swing symptoms. The caregiver turned to her and said: "Sometimes she's *just a-layin' there miseryin'* [feeling bad/depressed] and other times she's got the *allovers* [nervousness] (adapted from Flan, 1991, p. 135).

African Americans may also primarily use English. However, when the practitioner enters their diverse ethnic domain, it must be recognized that the ethnic group members have distinct systems of linguistic communication with unique displays of English.

> Case 1.2. The provider interviewed the African American caregiver in her home, in a rural area that formed part of the dementia program's service catchment area. The caregiver

described her aunt's dementing condition as a problem of having *high blood,* a colloqui-alism at times used by more traditional, culture-oriented older African Americans to de-scribe dementing illness (Gaines, 1988–1989). This phraseology may be less common at present, now that some information about Alzheimer's disease and related disorders has begun to extend to this ethnic population.

In addition to spoken or written language, it is important to keep in mind that an ethnic group's communication system includes its artwork and preferred decorative household artifacts; the observance of historical events and special holidays; and the key people, past or present, who are held up as models of respect or reverence by the group as a whole. Through careful attention, the observant professional or provider can pick up on these features of group life fairly quickly.

The second characteristic of ethnicity centers around the shared interactional pat-terns of the group members as well as their customs. These relational patterns are most often reflected in the way marital, familial, and core friendships are maintained. In the current literature these types of associations are known as *primary group* or *ingroup* ties (Bates & Babchuck, 1961; C. Cooley, 1909; Farris, 1932; Gudykunst, 1994; Litwak & Szelenyi, 1969; Popenoe, 1971; Valle, 1985; Valle & Bensussen, 1986). These ties also continue over time and include a considerable amount of affec-tive (feeling type) content. For example, the relationship patterns spoken about here may include the "unconditional" pulling together of the ingroup ethnic group mem-bers when they are confronting outside influences—even where the group members might have underlying conflictual relationships with each other. In this circumstance, group bonds are often expressed in powerful ways, bordering on what can be called self-centered, or *ethnocentric* orientations. Overall, ingroup bonds remain strong rallying points for the ethnically linked members and usually take some effort on the part of the practitioner to both decipher and penetrate.

The third aspect of ethnicity rests in the shared values and normative expectations of specific cultural groups. Understanding the role of these cultural elements requires some advance knowledge and skill on the part of the practitioner. This area is the most subtle of the three clusters of characteristics that define ethnic groups (Gudykunst, 1994; Valle, 1990a, 1994). The values arena is generally the least clearly in evidence at the initial meetings between the professional or provider and the ethnically diverse client. The reason for this is that, for the most part, values and beliefs are very privately held. They are not worn on the outside of relationships, so to speak, but rather form a pattern of *ethnocultural veils* (Fegurgur, 1995; Henderson & Gutierrez-Mayka, 1992; Valle, 1990a), which the practitioner must pull aside on an ongoing basis.

Most often, values and beliefs must be inferred from the statements and actions of the members of a specific ethnic group. Values and beliefs set the tone about how people are expected to act toward each other, even within one's own ethnic group, especially if they are strangers to each other (Gudykunst, 1994). They also contribute to the meaning given to specific situations in which people find themselves. Values and beliefs are also based on individuals' personal experiences, which are usually accumulated over a lifetime and which are lived in the context of their primary refer-ence groups, which include the family and the ethnic group as a whole. However, from the direct practice standpoint a further clarification about the values arena is indicated. Sometimes a person's values and behaviors do not coincide exactly. As practitioners are aware, there may be inner conflicts, or there may be pressures from outside sources, all of which can influence the more "idealized" aspects of individual or ethnic group values. The concept of *cognitive dissonance* is often used to indicate the gap between inner attitudes or beliefs and actual behaviors (Festinger, 1962).

Therefore, in addressing the values area of ethnic group life, the professional or provider must move slowly in attempting to understand the meaning that specific events and issues have for the target ethnic group members. For example, the practitioner has to be on guard against making assumptions that what is being said about Alzheimer's disease and related dementias from the medical or scientific standpoint is actually understood by the ethnically diverse client (Rogler, 1993). The professional or provider may be making quite different interpretations from the ones the client is making about the problems or solutions being addressed. Additionally, the practitioner must not expect immediate or total follow-through between suggested careplan actions and actual ethnically diverse client behaviors, especially where culturally held attitudes or beliefs may intervene.

> Case 1.3. Mr. Kataga had been diagnosed as having Alzheimer's disease. The doctor, who had known Mr. Kataga for a number of years, as they had both participated in Japanese American Civic League activities together, saw him as possibly benefiting from a day care program. He suggested this to Mrs. Kataga. The doctor's nurse, with the wife's approval, made an appointment for the couple to visit the dementia day care program at the Japanese Social Service Center. It soon became clear to the intake social worker at the center that Mrs. Kataga had come to the appointment to please the doctor. She had no real desire to place Mr. Kataga, as she felt it was her wifely duty to care for him at home as long as she could. She asked her son to communicate to the doctor her appreciation for his suggestion and his friendship with her husband.

When the issue had been discussed and the appointment had been made, it even appeared to the doctor, a fellow Japanese American, that Mrs. Kataga was in agreement to bring her husband to the dementia day care program. On closer analysis, however, she actually was following through with courtesy expressed to a person in authority. Her real wishes were quite different. The Japanese social service intake worker, with experience and knowledge about similar situations, had sufficient time to be able to understand Mrs. Kataga's true views and assisted her to establish a different program of home care assistance.

Universality of Culture and Ethnicity

An additional clarification about the notions of ethnicity and culture is in order at this point in the discussion. The examples to be provided throughout this text will most often refer to groups whose ethnocultural orientations are distinct from the more mainstream, U.S. English-speaking or Euro-Anglo–based society. In fact, it is this latter group that will be referred to as representing the *mainstream culture,* or *umbrella* or *host society* throughout the narrative (Samovar & Porter, 1995). However, the designation of mainstream culture is itself an oversimplification of the notion of ethnicity and culture and has to be understood in a more pluralistic sense. The phrase glosses over the very real diversity present in host or mainstream society through its Anglo-ethnic subgroups (Gelfand & Fandetti, 1980; Hraba, 1994; Keith et al., 1994; Kromkowski, 1993–1994; McLemore, 1994; M. Novak, 1972; Pedraza & Rumbaut, 1996). For example, the elderly patient from central Iowa, the caregiver from eastern Massachusetts, and the dementia-affected family from south Texas all come with long-standing diverse regional cultural orientations. There are also noticeable regional language differences (McLemore, 1994). Another way to look at mainstream society's cultural differences is to observe the generational differences with regard to interactional styles and normative expectations that practitioners often encounter among all cultures (Clark & Anderson, 1967; Sokolovsky, 1990).

Therefore, professionals and providers must be alert to the presence of distinct ethnicities among the mainstream groups—even if these "ethnic" differences might be based on generationally enculturated experiences or local regional variations (Clark & Anderson, 1967; Gelfand & Fandetti, 1980). Different eras imprint different value perspectives on the people who have lived through them (Green, 1987). Practitioners, therefore, must guard against making very broad stereotypic assumptions even about mainstream culture clients. Just because the practitioner and client seemingly speak the same style of English does not mean it is correct to assume that both are talking from the same value–belief point of reference. The supposition that all share the same perceptions about the world is simply not so.

> Case 1.4. Mrs. Arnold, now 85 and of Anglo heritage, came to a residential setting after long years of living alone in Georgia after the death of her husband. She was semi-immobilized by her osteoporosis and her severe arthritis and was unable to perform many of the bending-over and picking-up and room cleaning tasks for herself. However, she was very disturbed at the way the cleaning staff came through her room and were handling her personal items as they dusted or moved them around as they cleaned. She complained at a resident council meeting: "The cleaning ladies do a good job of dusting and mopping, but some of my things are very private. This wasn't the way I cleaned when I helped my mother when she was ill. I always asked mother: 'Can I clean the top of your dressing table?' Where are people's manners nowadays, anyway?".

Certainly, the residential cleaning staff meant well, but they had overlooked a seemingly small, yet very real expectation on the part of Mrs. Arnold. There are many other "ethnic" considerations that have been inappropriately homogenized when working with elderly members from the host society's ethnic groups. It is not only that local idiomatic expressions are ignored but also that important subtleties around help-giving and help-accepting, as well as expectations about what constitutes proper conduct between strangers, are lost.

For example, do older residents of Euro-Anglo heritage in skilled-nursing facilities really like to be called by their first names any more than Latinos or Asian Americans do? Are non-English–speaking ethnics the only ones who have formal and informal personal pronouns in their vocabulary? Although the pronoun *you* in English can be applied in both a formal and informal context, the non-alert practitioner might miss the interpersonal exchange expectations of Anglo heritage individuals from different generations. Many people whose youth dates to either the 1930's Depression era or the World War II period were brought up at a time when "Mr.," "Mrs.," and "Miss" were still ordinarily used when younger persons addressed older individuals. This same form of courtesy also prevailed when adults—who were strangers to each other—met initially to conduct business. Many older Euro-Anglo ethnics share this kind of "formal manners" cultural upbringing, and dementing illness may be locking them back within that period of their lives when they used these cultural subtleties. In the haste to expedite services, practitioners and service personnel may forget these considerations.

The overarching principle at work here is that everybody, whether from the mainstream–host society or from an ethnically diverse group, has an ethnicity. This principle holds regardless of whether individuals are explicitly aware of it. In brief, the ideas of culture and ethnicity need to be applied across the board to both mainstream and ethnically diverse groups (Grabowski & Franz, 1992–1993). However, the relevance of this recommendation might be better understood if explored first in the context of the experiences of ethnocultural populations that are linguistically, interactionally, and normatively distinct from the mainstream groups.

MULTICULTURAL VERSUS ETHNIC-SPECIFIC ORIENTATIONS

As a part of the multicultural environment (Song & Kim, 1993), service organizations and their personnel usually are active in areas where a great variety of ethnocultural groups reside (Alzheimer's Disease and Related Disorders Association, 1994; Braun, Takamura, Forman, Sasaki, & Meininger, 1995; Valle, 1988–1989). At the same time, requests for services are most often made by clients from specific ethnic groups. This fact brings with it the demand that the professional or provider demonstrate both multicultural alertness and intercultural engagement competence directed to specific ethnic groups. Therein arises a basic tension that may be felt by both the practitioner in the field and the reader of this text. However, a false dichotomy may perhaps be drawn here. Practitioners and their service organizations can be both multiculturally and ethnic-specific oriented.

First, to work effectively with ethnically diverse groups, the professional or provider must be specifically capable of engaging the ethnic client group asking for, or being targeted for, dementia-care services. This requires that the practitioner become knowledgeable about the ethnic group's specific cultural indicators. The group members will have their own language and communication requirements and will bring their unique culture-of-origin traditions and perspectives to the table. The practitioner has to be ready to respond to these unique patterns. At the same time, as noted earlier, dementing illness affects individuals and families of many different ethnic group affiliations. Therefore, the practitioner needs to also maintain a capability of responding to multiple requests for services coming from people of varied cultural backgrounds. In such instances practitioners who actually shift their style of approach to respond to different groups are, in effect, entering into the multicultural arena. Therefore, although this text will stress the need for the practitioner to develop ethnic-specific competencies, these skills must also be translated into a multicultural alertness.

DEVELOPMENT OF A CROSS-CULTURAL COMFORT ZONE

Admittedly, it is generally accurate to say that one is more comfortable with one's culture-of-origin. Therefore, the demand on the professional or provider to develop ethnic-specific capabilities while at the same time remaining ready to engage the multicultural reality in most, if not all, service environments, can generate stressors for the practitioner. It may be difficult at first to find one's comfort zone. In this regard, it should be noted that individuals who are bilingual and bicultural are able to extend their comfort zone to the two cultures that have influenced their lives. These bilingual/bicultural professionals or providers may also have an edge in being able to apply the principles related to ethnic-specific situations to the multicultural workplace potentially broadening their *intercultural engagement comfort zone.*

A possible strategy for the monocultural English-speaking professionals or providers to broaden their cross-cultural comfort zone is to team up in *bicultural-pairs.* As described beginning with Chapter 4 and in subsequent segments of the text, a monocultural practitioner in a bicultural-pair joins forces with a biculturally competent individual to bring dementia-care services to ethnically diverse populations. These and other notions, which have so far just been touched on, will be amplified throughout the delineation of the cultural mapping process in Part One.

REVIEW OF KEY WORKING ASSUMPTIONS

1. **There is an ethnically diverse population explosion at work throughout dementia-care service environments.** Practitioners and their parent organizations must broaden their outlooks to encompass the actual diversity present within their catchment areas. This revolution of diversity has been going on for some time. Although a diverse clientele may not be showing up regularly with reference to the current dementia-care service networks, providers need to examine their approaches for engaging ethnically diverse clients, who may have different, and more traditional, culture-of-origin understandings about dementing illness or who simply may not have heard about dementia-care services in a linguistic format intelligible to themselves and other members of their ethnic group.

2. **Dementing illness is making its presence felt within ethnically diverse populations.** The ravages of dementing illnesses are being experienced by ethnically diverse groups in the United States. There is a responsibility on the part of professionals and providers, as well as their parent organizations, to address the needs of these populations. This responsibility extends equally whether dementia-care needs are being directly manifested by the members of the ethnic groups or are being kept relatively hidden within the ethnic group's own processes. Neglect of these needs at any level is hurtful.

3. **There is an accompanying responsibility on the part of the dementia-care field to address the development of a culture-competent cadre of professionals and providers to meet the emerging needs diverse populations.** Actually, the responsibility for the development of intercultural com-

petency in the dementia-care arena rests on the shoulders of individual practitioners as well as those of their parent organizations. The models for developing intercultural engagement capabilities are readily available (Berghe, 1972; Butcher, 1982; Cushner & Brislin, 1996; Harris & Moran, 1987; Sue & Sue, 1990; Triandis, Bontempo, Leung, & Hui, 1990). One is presented in this text that is applicable at both the individual and organizational levels.

END NOTE: RECOGNITION OF ETHNICALLY DIVERSE GROUPS

A positive sign that some effort is underway can be noted in the increasing availability of culturally diverse information about a variety of ethnocultural groups. For example, one can find information about Alzheimer's disease and related dementing illness that encompasses ethnically diverse groups. Also, there is some key dementing illness information available for selected ethnic groups, such as Hispanics (Mace & Rabins, 1990; Powell & Courtice, 1990; Sizemore, Ochoa-Coover, West, & Mahon, 1991; Alzheimer's Cross Cultural Research and Development, 1992; Institute for Community Research, 1992; Gallagher-Thompson et al., 1992). There is material specific to Asian American populations (Braun et al., 1995) and to African Americans (*Alzheimer's: A family affair,* 1990). There also is additional information about ethnically diverse populations at both the national headquarters level of the Alzheimer's Association and at the local level from chapters of the association (Alzheimer's Disease and Related Disorders Association, 1994).

However, two problems present themselves with regard to the availability of culturally and linguistically pertinent information on dementing illness. The first is the *lack of timeliness* with which the most current basic information is communicated to ethnically diverse populations. Dissemination of vital information takes more of a catch-up approach, with the content appearing in the languages of ethnically diverse populations one to several years after becoming available in English. When advances are made in dementia-care strategies, or when medical and scientific breakthroughs occur, they are not routinely reported in languages appropriate for consumption by ethnically diverse groups in the United States—with the accent placed on *routinely.*

The second difficulty relates to the *lack of multicultural thoroughness* of the dissemination of existing dementing illness information in multiple language formats. This supply of available information has yet to permeate throughout the complete multiculturally varied dementia-affected communities in the same manner that the content is available in English.

The capability exists to address both problems. The business community has demonstrated the ease of information dissemination through its marketing apparatus. One need only travel throughout ethnically diverse neighborhoods to see the advertisements that abound as well as the information in different languages about specific products. It would appear that an analogous approach can be taken with respect to dementing illness. The public health field likewise can point to informational content for varied ethnocultural groups around many specific health topics. These are the places to start.

Chapter 2

Culture and the Acculturation Continuum

It is universally recognized that Alzheimer's disease not only ravages the individual but has a devastating impact on the dementia-affected person's caregiving network. However, what is less recognized is that the caregiving network responds in cultural ways stemming from the network members' ethnic group orientations (Gaines, 1988–1989; Henderson & Gutierrez-Mayka, 1992; Valle, 1981, 1989, 1994). In facilitating the care network's coping responses, therefore, it is crucial that the professional or provider understand the role culture may play within the caregiving response patterns encountered (Havenaar, 1990; Jecker, Carrese, & Pearlman, 1995; Jenkins & Karno; 1992; Krause & Wray, 1991; Lin, Innui, Kleirman, & Womak, 1982; Mauro, Sato, & Tucker, 1992; Mesquita & Frijda, 1992; Szapocznik & Kurtines, 1993). To this end, then, the professional or provider needs not only to develop a profile of the dementing condition but also to actively engage in culturally mapping the situation that is encountered.

A suggested starting point for the overall cultural mapping process is for the professional or provider to develop a thorough understanding of the notion of culture itself. The discussion that follows is designed to give the practitioner access to cultural concepts relevant to assessment and intervention activities with ethnically diverse populations. In addition, the notion of an *acculturation continuum* is presented. This aspect of cultural theory accepts the ongoing adaptation of the culture of origin that people bring with them. The acculturation continuum concept has particular application to ethnic populations residing within a host society such as the United States, where cultural assimilation takes place unevenly (Montalvo & Gutierrez, 1989).

The cultural mapping discussion below also highlights how important it is that the practitioner be able to appropriately distinguish social status factors such as income, education, and literacy levels and sort them from the key descriptors of culture, namely, language, customs, and beliefs.

DIFFICULTIES WITH THE NOTION OF CULTURE

First, to the busy professional or provider, the concept of culture might appear as very abstract and subject to a host of interpretations and definitions (Agar, 1994). To a large extent the abstract aspects of culture arise because, generally speaking, culture is not always consciously seen (Cushner & Brislin, 1996). Rather, what is actually experienced is people behaving according to sets of rules that are not always clear to the observer (Banks, 1995). In other instances a culture's products may be experienced in ways that are enjoyed at the feeling level rather than evaluated cognitively. Examples can include a culture's music, its cuisine, and its festivals. Here the observer may not be paying explicit attention to the cultural dimension of the experience but rather enjoying the moment without recognizing the historical and value-laden implications of the events themselves. It is true that cultures have features that are obviously visible. At the same time they are also full of less visible undercurrents (Brownlee, 1978, p. v). In this context, most people, whether professionals, providers, or community residents, tend to live their everyday lives without being consciously alert to their own or others' underlying assumptions about the world (Brownlee, 1978, pp. 245–246). In this context they tend to act unconsciously from their own ethnocentric value orientations (Ivey, 1994, p. 4).

Second, what also makes it difficult to come to grips with the notion of culture is that it is not a stationary phenomenon. From the outside, a culture, or an ethnic group, might give the appearance of being fixed in another time and place, especially when the practitioner runs into traditional outlooks based on culture-of-origin perspectives that are different from those of U.S. mainstream society (Cowgill, 1986). The reality is quite different. Traditional outlooks persist over time, but as Cowgill (p. 4) indicates, changes from outside influences also enter into the picture of the ethnically diverse family group, although the rate or degree of such change may be quite different for individuals or different ethnic groups as a whole. This is very much the situation of the ethnically diverse populations residing within the U.S. host society. The culture that group members brought with them at the point of their first arrival will have undergone alteration regardless of the reasons for which they first immigrated (Cheng, 1987, p. 9). This often takes place behind the scenes, as there is much interaction between the ethnic group members and the host society that goes unrecorded. For example, English words or expressions start to enter the languages of different ethnic groups, expressed in what is often called *code switching,* which indicates the use or borrowing of terms from different languages (Arámbula, 1992; Hamayan

& Damico, 1991; Hyltenstam & Obler, 1989; Mattes & Omark, 1984). Customs of the host culture become internalized within the ethnocultural group. The reality of these almost imperceptible changes in the original culture hit home very clearly to bicultural individuals who return to the locales where their families originated. As a case in point, Latinos from the United States who visit their countries of origin often hear how *agringado* (Americanized) they have become. African Americans who visit parts of Africa do find their roots, but they also find that their own ethnic identity differs from that of ethnocultural groups now residing in their locale of origin. These people, returning to their homelands after the passage of only a single generation, often find that they straddle two worlds (Grosjean, 1982; Pedraza & Rumbaut, 1996).

The malleability of culture also is visible with regard to the U.S. host society itself. Ethnically diverse groups in turn have an impact on the broader society. The simple exercise of examining the Yellow Pages in almost any region of the United States will reveal a wide selection of uniquely ethnic restaurants. The regular telephone directories can likewise reveal a wide range of ethnic surnames in much greater quantities than was found two decades ago, reflecting the worldwide context of immigration patterns to this country since World War II.

The fluid qualities of culture can be noted in all of these areas, but so can the culture's more enduring, or static, aspects. For example, when health problems and service needs arise among the more traditional-culture–oriented ethnic group members, the professional or provider very often encounters coping attitudes and practices that may appear quite unrelated to what is known about dementing illness from current medical or scientific investigation. Ethnic family members operating from a *notion of shame* may well try to hide the elder's dementia until the problems reach catastrophic proportions (Elliot et al., 1996). In other instances, Alzheimer's disease may be attributed to causes rooted in folk beliefs. At the same time, the practitioner may come across some family members from the ethnically diverse group vainly trying to contact the mainstream service organizations for help with their problems, but not being successful because of the underlying cultural misunderstandings involved (Brownlee, 1978).

It is at this point of contact where breakdowns occur between the culturally diverse client and the English-speaking monocultural professional or provider. These breakdowns take place especially when the practitioner is unprepared to address the impact of culture (Brownlee, 1978). Because of the intensity of the care needs that sometimes accompany dementing illness situations, it can happen that professionals or practitioners will find their attention diverted away from cultural concerns. Under these circumstances it usually takes that face-to-face contact with someone else's cultural expectations, namely, the ethnically diverse client's distinctly different cultural outlooks, before the professional or provider becomes directly aware of the reality of the cultural diversity present in the dementia-care situation.

However, more is required of the cross-culturally competent practitioner. It is most important that the professional or provider avoids having cultural considerations enter the dementia assessment or careplanning situation by happenstance. From a cross-cultural practice/intercultural engagement perspective, this approach is not acceptable. What is required is that professionals and providers who are engaged in offering ethnically diverse dementia care give priority to acquiring an up-front understanding of the ethnically diverse client's cultural orientations. Time and effort have to be given to planning ahead for the cultural input to the dementia assessment. The practitioner has to anticipate the cultural dimensions of the contact that will take place (Brownlee, 1978). The clear implication is that the incorporation of cultural assessment capabilities into the practitioner's repertoire of knowledge and skills will greatly enhance dementia-care service to ethnically diverse populations.

GAINING A WORKING UNDERSTANDING OF CULTURE

A number of practical approaches can be used for gaining cross-cultural or intercultural understanding. The core of the *cultural mapping strategy* is summarized here and outlined in greater depth throughout the succeeding chapters of Part One. A crucial step forward for professionals and providers is to get outside of their own "cultural world" and to engage ethnically diverse populations in the context of theirs (Agar, 1994). However, it is important to recognize that cultural understanding will not arrive simply by experience alone. Family members will not bring books with them outlining their ethnic orientations. Moreover, ethnically diverse families will not be ready to enter provider systems just because the agency personnel have goodwill toward them, or even because they are eligible for a specific service. Most likely the ethnically diverse family members/significant others caring for a dementia-affected elder will be driven by the crisis in which they find themselves. However, the ethnic client group members will be looking to make sense of what is available, what they can actually access, and what is offered by professionals and providers in the context of their informational as well as their values–belief and normative-understandings basepoint.

Practitioners, especially professionals and providers in the dementing illness arena, therefore, need to ingrain in themselves the awareness that cross-cultural or intercultural understanding demands conceptual preparation on their part before they rush out to engage in outreach and service delivery (Adams, 1980; Alzheimer's Disease and Related Disorders Association, 1994; N. B. Anderson & Cohen, 1989). Dementia-centered service and research organizations would not consider sending staff out into the field or into the clinic unprepared to work with the complexities of Alzheimer's disease and related disorders. Courses are offered. Training is provided. A conceptual and informational competency about dementing illness and its impact on the brain and on behavior is required. Why, then, should it be any different with respect to approaching the complexities of cultural intervention? The business management field already has been engaged in cross-cultural training for a number of years (Harris & Moran, 1987; Fine, 1995). Why can't the dementia-care arena do the same?

It is understood that such a concerted approach to intercultural work is difficult to put into practice. Economic constraints and the shortage of available bilingual/bicultural personnel put very real pressures on provider systems and has them operating on a different "cultural" track. For example, the mainstream cultural approach, without stating it, has its service systems organized so that the consumer finds and learns to use particular programs. There may be some outreach and community or consumer education. There may even be a hurried search for consumers when the census is down, or when the research subject quotas are not met. However, the core value orientation of the existing dementia organizational systems, regardless of whether they are diagnostic clinics, day centers, or skilled nursing facilities, is to have consumers become familiar with them and their functions rather than the other way around.

This agency "cultural bias" is not easily recognized or overcome (Brownlee, 1978). To do so, professionals or providers generally have to step outside of their own cognitive and emotional home base. They have to leave the relative comfort of their own formal training backgrounds to see their own service organizations through the eyes of very needy but interculturally confused individuals and family groups coming for help. When viewing their organization from this perspective, the professional or practitioner can understand how the agency's formal and informal communications, its normative procedures, and its underlying philosophy can be totally misunderstood by the ethnically diverse person who is lost in a maze of misunderstood signals.

All of these considerations are not intended to sidetrack the main direction of the discussion at hand. However, the difficulties must be acknowledged in proceeding to develop an understanding of the role of culture and of attaining a cross-cultural practice capability. Whatever the impediments, a conceptual framework must be developed so that the practitioner or provider can understand the dementia-affected person's culture of origin. This is seen as especially true where the damage to brain tissue by most dementing conditions forces the affected person farther and farther back into his or her long-term memory, where the culture-of-origin orientations still reside. The family members seeking to accommodate the dementia-affected elder are likewise forced back into this more traditional cultural orientation, as are practitioners.

Case 2.1. The bilingual/bicultural Latino practitioner had been working for some time with the Chavez family. The elder Mrs. Chavez had been diagnosed with Alzheimer's disease. Her caregiver husband had recently died, and the primary caregiving role had fallen to the oldest daughter, Alma. As a fellow bilingual professional in the allied field of child welfare, Alma understood service programs quite well, but out of respect to her deceased father's traditional views she was considering working part time as an alternative to not enrolling her mother in a day care program. As Alma said, "I know such programs are good. I often recommend them to people on my caseload, but I feel a responsibility to my heritage. Papa would not have approved my abandoning Mamá."

ACCULTURATION MODEL

To approach the intercultural engagement process, it is helpful to combine both the fixed and the fluid qualities of culture into a single formulation. The Chavez case, Case 2.1 (above), demonstrates both the fixed aspects of culture—namely, Alma's desire to respect her deceased father's wishes—and the fluid nature of new or acquired professional cultural input in that, as a practitioner, she could readily make referrals to services for her own clients. In this manner, when one is looking at the quiltwork of ethnically diverse groups and individuals within the broader U.S. society, the professional or provider can capture all the pertinent cultural aspects relating to the dementing illness situation being observed. Alma could be engaged with professional understandings with regard to her practitioner role; however, she needs to be reached in her innermost cultural core with reference to her caregiver role. It is evident that culture has the potential for lifetime permanence in some respects as well as the ability to be modified over time in other respects (Agar, 1994; Szapocznik & Kurtines, 1993; Valle, 1990a, 1994; Westermeyer, 1987).

From the professional's or the provider's standpoint, a conceptual strategy that can be used to capture the seemingly contradictory aspects of the cultural experience is to apply the acculturation continuum model. Through the use of the acculturation continuum framework, the professional or provider can account for: (a) the traditional outlooks and behaviors within specific ethnocultural groups and their members, (b) the bicultural elements of the family or ethnic group being targeted for dementia-related services, and (c) the acculturated behaviors and attitudes of individuals and of the group as a whole. Figure 2.1 summarizes the model.

The principle of acculturation proposes that ethnic group members are influenced consciously or unconsciously, directly or indirectly, by living within a host society (Betancourt & Regeser López, 1993; Cuellar, Arnold, & Maldonado, 1995; Cuellar, Harris, & Jasso, 1980; Smart & Smart, 1993; Szapocznik & Kurtines, 1993). This means that at any point in time some of the members of a specific ethnic group may lean in the direction of being more traditional in their outlooks, that is to say, more linked to their culture-of-origin. Other members may be more bicultural and may take their cues from both their traditional culture and the host society in which they live. Still other members of the same ethnic group may have accommodated themselves much more to the host social environment. In essence, they have become *acculturated* to the mainstream society (Valle, 1994). The professional or provider must be ready to encounter the full spectrum of the acculturation continuum in almost any situation, whether it involves a family as a whole or the family's individual members. Moreover, in the context of the range of possibilities, some group members may have settled on one point in the continuum; for example, they may be more traditional in their outlooks, whereas others will have become more acculturated to the host society.

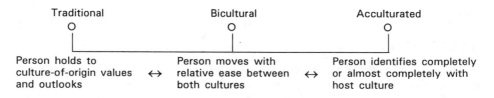

Figure 2.1 Acculturation continuum framework.

Case 2.2. By telephone, the practitioner set up an initial session to develop a cultural–historical case profile of the Martin family. During the dementia assessment process she noted that the grandfather was expressing himself in English mixed with Spanish, although no mention had been previously made about a specific ethnocultural heritage. Further probing revealed that the dementia-affected Mr. Martin had changed the family name from Martinez to Martin earlier in his life so that the family could have better opportunities. English became the household language. The grandchildren now no longer spoke Spanish or related to the older family traditions. However, the surfacing of Mr. Martin's primary language as his dementia progressed now posed an acculturation barrier for the careplan. The practitioner realized that the family would need to be communicated with in English, whereas Mr. Martin would require bilingual communication, with the probability that eventually monolingual Spanish language services would be required.

First, the literature makes it clear that ethnic groups evolve over time whether they desire to or not, as in the Martin case (Case 2.2). Moreover, on a worldwide basis, there is clear evidence that even the more isolated human groups adopt some of the tools, artifacts, and customs of more technologically oriented societies. Second, as noted earlier, ethnic groups, especially in the United States, exist as part of a host society that influences their values and their interactions in real ways. This makes them even more prone to acculturation influences in succeeding generations. Third, there is an equally strong countervailing force within very strongly traditional ethnic groups to preserve aspects of their authentic primary cultural group orientations (McLemore, 1994) in the context of residual values maintained by ethnically diverse group members (Valle, 1990b). The literature documents a rise in ethnic consciousness throughout the United States and an accompanying pull among the third-, fourth, and even more distant generation members of ethnic groups to return to many of their traditional ways (McLemore, 1994). The Native American/American Indian group is only one example of this "ethnic revival" trend.

CASE 2.3. Carl had revived the tribal family name of Bearclaw. He had begun to incorporate traditional Cheyenne ceremonies into the family's daily life. Now that serious memory problems had affected his grandmother since her stroke, Carl spent much more time with his grandfather to learn more of the tribal customs and traditions. Carl's wife and the children enjoyed participating in the ceremonies. The grandmother likewise took pleasure from the same events.

The earlier Martin case (Case 2.2) presents a move by a family group to accommodate the host society, whereas the Bearclaw case (Case 2.3) provides a contrast, in that the whole family is returning to their traditional ethnic ways, thereby accommodating not only their own needs but those of the dementia-affected family member as well. The usefulness of the acculturation model, therefore, is that it can not only be used flexibly but that it can also be made to apply to an ethnic group as a whole, to a family, or to specific individuals. Of special importance is that the model allows the professional or practitioner to track client outlooks and behaviors in a variety of settings, such as at home, at the workplace, or in the general community. In each of these circumstances, the ethnic group as a whole, families as a subgroup, or individuals can at times be found to occupy different *cultural spaces*. For example, different members of an ethnic group may have immigrated at different points in time. Some of the elderly ethnic group members, having immigrated as children, may be quite far away in time from their original home culture. Different ethnic group members may also demonstrate different skill levels in mastering the host society's language and customs. Others will be monolingual in their own traditional language, whereas still others, who may identify more with their traditional culture, may nonetheless have lost their ability to speak their own traditional language.

It is vital for the practitioner to have a tool to grasp the considerable cultural variation within the ranks of any single ethnic group. By looking at ethnic groups in terms of seeing their lives taking place along an acculturation continuum, the practitioner can gain an understanding of actions and attitudes that might otherwise appear to be anomalies. These considerations become very important with respect to conducting a comprehensive assessment of dementing illness with members of ethnically diverse populations. These understandings are likewise important when it comes to designing and subsequently implementing careplans. For instance, as the dementing disorder of Alzheimer's disease progresses, the dementia-affected elder may have lost more recently learned information, such as the ability to speak English (Arámbula, 1992), or the ability to handle more mainstream cultural experiences. The elder's perceptions may now reside within the cultural place of his or her youth. All secondarily learned cultural accommodation skills have been wiped away. Recognition of these dimensions of patient and family functioning is as essential to the overall evaluation and treatment plan as the other parts of differential diagnostic process.

Putting the Acculturation Model into Practice

In putting the acculturation continuum framework into practice, the professional or provider needs to be certain to conduct the comprehensive cultural assessment in a timely manner. Undertaking a cultural assessment concurrently within the differential diagnostic evaluation for dementia is highly recommended. However, because of a variety of circumstances outside the immediate control of the individual practitioner, it can happen that the cultural assessment and the dementia assessment will be undertaken separately. Some reasons for this have been alluded to earlier in the text, particularly with regard to the possible indifference of many existing provider systems, the ever-present short supply of interculturally capable personnel, and the unavailability of funding. It can also happen that the costs of a full diagnostic evaluation might not be covered by the ethnically diverse family member's health care policy— this is to say, only determined medical procedures and treatments are covered. In other cases the cross-cultural evaluation resources simply may not be available.

Regardless of these circumstances, the professional and provider alike need to consider that the ethnically diverse patient and the family members are nonetheless owed an assessment that incorporates the cultural dimension. The health professional or provider may have to go to somewhat greater lengths to implement the cultural assessment. Without this component, a fully adequate, let alone appropriate, differential evaluation for dementing illness or treatment plan cannot ensue. For example, any assessment or treatment plan encompassing the key activities of daily living (ADLs;

such as feeding, toileting, bathing, etc.) or the more instrumental activities of daily living (IADLs; such as transportation, arranging financial and legal matters, etc.) calls for a cultural assessment input. Basically, help-engaging activities involving ethnically diverse groups place the professional or provider squarely into the members' cultural pathways (Rogler & Cortes, 1993). Therefore, a specifically focused cultural assessment becomes an integral part of a true comprehensive diagnostic assessment and treatment plan.

In proceeding to make the cultural assessment, the initial step is to become alert to the importance of language and communication patterns. In practical terms it might be useful to keep in mind that ethnically diverse family members, particularly those for whom English is a second language, may attach very different cultural meanings to what is being communicated about Alzheimer's disease and dementing illness (Yeo et al., 1996). This can happen even if English is being used, because they will be using their native language as a point of reference. For example, the professional or provider may be focusing on the neurological aspects of Alzheimer's disease, whereas the family members, given their lack of knowledge, may be associating the changes that have taken place in the elder's behavior to cultural or spiritual beliefs, which leads them to seek corresponding ethnocultural remedies.

Case 2.4. The Haitian bilingual/bicultural practitioner had asked for the opportunity for a home conference to explain the nature of Alzheimer's disease. The elder Mr. Maurice, a 78-year-old refugee Haitian American patient, had just received a diagnosis at the clinic, and some confusions had arisen within the family. Mrs. Maurice felt that her husband should be taken to Haiti for spiritual treatment to take away a possible spell that was producing his out-of-character behavior.

The practitioner began a three-pronged approach. First, she recognized that the pull of the homeland cultural beliefs was strong for Mrs. Maurice. However, even though some political stability had come to Haiti, she wanted to be sure that Mrs. Maurice would be able to continue to live there and fully care for her husband. Second, the practitioner needed to know if Mrs. Maurice wanted to return to Haiti permanently or just to obtain spiritual treatment for her husband. If Mrs. Maurice wanted to return for the spiritual treatment, the practitioner was ready to suggest alternative ceremonies available within the U.S. Haitian community. Last, she also wanted to provide the medical and clinical facts of dementing illness, and the brain damage that accompanies Alzheimer's disease, to give Mrs. Maurice a well-rounded understanding of what the future would hold even after the spiritual support was obtained. The practitioner realized she would have to bridge the medical understanding of dementia by using some of the Haitian spiritual and common-day language.

It is important to keep in mind that sometimes the family member's native language does not have terms that are directly equivalent to the technical aspects of specialized dementia care service (Valle, 1994, pp. 33–34). In other instances, even if there are technical terms in the native language, the ethnic group family members may not have been exposed to them. Therefore, in preparing to communicate in the language of a specific ethnocultural group about such conditions as Alzheimer's disease, it is important to work toward finding culturally equivalent and understandable content, as the practitioner did in the Maurice case (Case 2.4). Moreover, the practitioner neither ignored nor overmagnified the Maurice family's search for spiritual treatment. Rather, this aspect of the intervention was handled as an integral component of the overall careplan.

A second sector in the cultural assessment that requires attention is the potentially different expectations about the *style* of the interaction that is considered appropriate by the target ethnic group members, especially what is considered appropriate within the family and with strangers. In addition to relating to the identified primary caregiver, it is vital to know if there are key secondary decision makers within the extended family who also have to be brought into the planned intercultural contacts (Bedolla, 1995). The practitioner needs to determine in what ways these significant others have to be consulted regarding the proposed planned care. From the family's standpoint there may also be unvoiced, but nonetheless expected, cultural protocols, that is, the target ethnic group's normal interactional expectatons, relating to home visits by professionals and providers as well as for clinical or residential setting visitations. For instance, it could be that the presence of multiple-generation family members is the norm for the ethnic group. If so, home visits may include quite large numbers of people, who could also be bringing their toddlers along. There could be an underlying expectation that these significant others will not be excluded from the clinical or residential setting visits. It is also not uncommon among many ethnic groups to incorporate non-blood relatives into the family (Gaines, 1988–1989). This means that at times family friends, informally adopted individuals, and even neighbors may be included in the family constellation of the dementia-affected elder. This is why it is so important to know the ethnic group's interactional style beforehand.

A third element of the cultural assessment is the documentation of the values and beliefs held by the ethnic group members around dementing illness, and particularly about going public, that is, going outside the family circle about what is happening with the elderly family member. This arena is even more subtle than the preceding items discussed, because values and beliefs are held within the person and can generally be seen only indirectly in the form of expressed attitudes, expectations, and orientations. However, careful preparatory work may help concretize the provider's approaches to these less tangible aspects of the ethnocultural heritage of the ethnically diverse dementia-affected elder and the caregiver.

As noted earlier, consideration of these multiple factors may bring varying degrees of discomfort to the practitioner, or possibly to the practitioner's parent organization, as they may be operating from the perspective of their professional cultures. However, the routine incorporation of these factors into the dementia evaluation process is essential to the appropriate assessment of ethnically diverse populations.

FACTORS OFTEN CONFUSED WITH CULTURE

There is still one additional step required to make the acculturation continuum–cultural assessment model fully workable. It is important to keep in mind that everything that has happened to the ethnically diverse group members is not, strictly speaking, cultural. Therefore, in addition to the cultural dimension, the professional or provider must be able to sort out the noncultural factors (Talamantes, Cornell, Espino, Lichtenstein, & Hazuda, 1996; Triandis et al., 1990). These include: (a) differentiating the *socioeconomic level* of the elder and of the caregiving social network from cultural attributes; (b) distinguishing the relative *social status* of the family and the ethnic group members from the core of their ethnicity; (c) isolating the residual effects of *prejudice* and *discrimination* from cultural outlooks; and (d) separating the caregiver's, the family members', and the elder's *levels of literacy* from cultural considerations.

Many ethnic groups within the U.S. host society are still in an underclass position. That is to say, the members of the ethnic group are less able, or completely unable, to have their voices heard or their needs met relative to influencing societal political and policy processes. They experience a greater scarcity of service resources, particularly with reference to dementing illness. Moreover, even when such resources are made available, they may not be easily accessible. This state of being resource poor can range from lacking of transportation through to the fact that the service resource, however culturally appropriate, is economically out of reach (Wallace, 1990). In addition, the ethnically diverse family members and the dementia-affected elder may have been the recipients of discriminatory actions both recently as well as earlier in their lives. These experiences may have long-term effects on the ethnic group members. In both of these instances the problems of linking to and using services may be not cultural in origin, but rather reflective of the member's overall social status.

Literacy also can play an equally important role, apart from culture, regarding the interactions of ethnically diverse groups and provider systems (Poplin & Phillips, 1993), especially in the area of dementing illness (Valle, 1994). No matter how culturally relevant the intended message has been made, it still may be delivered in a format that is beyond the skills of the target audience, particularly among the older, first-generation immigrant ethnic group members. Formal schooling may not have been a part of the ethnic group member's life experience—and if schooling was provided, it may have been very limited.

At the same time these characteristics are discussed with reference to ethnically diverse groups, it is important to avoid stereotyping. For example, the label of illiteracy cannot be applied across the board to all ethnically diverse populations. Literacy levels will vary from group to group as well as from member to member. Even though English may be new to them, some ethnocultural groups have native literate traditions that antedate those of European heritage groups. Chinese and Japanese Americans, as well as Indian Americans from the subcontinent of India itself, are exemplars of such traditions. Still others come from backgrounds based more on oral history. In actual everyday practice, literacy presents as a much more mixed picture. A priori assumptions, without supporting evidence, cannot be made about any ethnic group or individual from the group. A caregiver coming from a more literate culture may not be formally schooled, whereas another caregiver coming from a culture that emphasizes oral tradition may in fact be quite advanced with regard to formal schooling. With this said, however, it must be recognized that literacy, or perhaps better stated, *functional literacy,* namely, the ability to comprehend written content and to communicate in a written mode, may be more scarce in the general adult and aging world than many practitioners recognize. A recent study titled *Adult Literacy in*

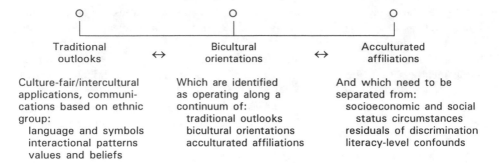

Figure 2.2 Acculturation model in full.

America (U.S. Department of Education, 1993) estimates that approximately 48% of the general (mainstream) U.S. population has functional literacy problems. Moreover, lower schooling levels, apart from dementing illness itself, is a problem within the current pre-World War II, age 65+ generation as a whole.

The relationship of the literacy issue to the dementing illness arena is that often the intake forms that are used, and the assessment measures that are applied (such as cognitive screens and neuropsychological tests), along with formal communications that are generally sent to families, may be missing the mark—even when the native language of the recipient is accommodated. The communication may be technically beyond the comprehension of the target ethnically diverse and even mainstream culture family group.

Figure 2.2 takes these cultural assessment distorting factors into account and presents a more complete view of the cultural assessment–acculturation continuum model. In this manner the elements that can be appropriately attributed to culture are identified. Those that may relate to the ethnically diverse client group's economic or social status can be disentangled. Both sets of factors—the cultural and the social status indicators—are important. They are often intertwined in the real world situation of the ethnically diverse client; however, they belong to different domains of the assessment being made, and for analytical purposes they need to be kept separate.

LINKING THE MODEL TO DEMENTING ILLNESS

For the dementia-care practitioner there is still one more link to make: namely, the application of the fully delineated cultural assessment framework to dementing illness. As Valle (1990a) suggests, the professional or provider approaching the culturally diverse dementing illness assessment situation would operate along a dual axis, as outlined in Figure 2.3. The different aspects of the clinical differential diagnostic evaluation that seek to identify both the kind and the extent of the patient's dementing condition along with the stress and burden felt by the caregivers/family members are grouped along the vertical axis. The cultural component of the evaluation can be seen along the horizontal axis and, as indicated throughout the discussion above, the professional or provider needs to be cognizant of the fact that the client group members will express their ethnicity along the acculturation continuum as detailed.

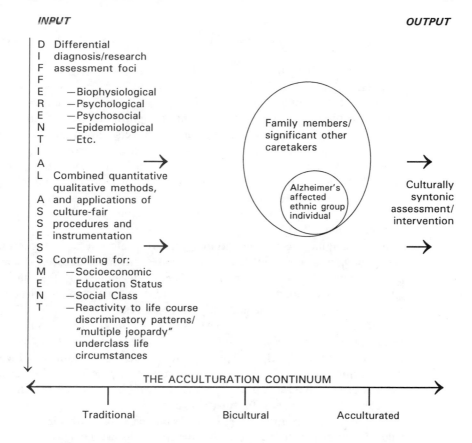

INPUT   *OUTPUT*

D Differential
I   diagnosis/research
F assessment foci
F
E   —Biophysiological
R   —Psychological
E   —Psychosocial
N   —Epidemiological
T   —Etc.
I
A
L   Combined quantitative
     qualitative methods,
A and applications of
S culture-fair
S procedures and
E instrumentation
S
S Controlling for:
M   —Socioeconomic
E   Education Status
N   —Social Class
T   —Reactivity to life course
          discriminatory patterns/
          "multiple jeopardy"
          underclass life
          circumstances

Family members/
significant other
caretakers

Alzheimer's
affected
ethnic group
individual

Culturally
syntonic
assessment/
intervention

THE ACCULTURATION CONTINUUM

Traditional   Bicultural   Acculturated

ASSESSED IN TERMS OF:

 • Communication patterns (language and symbols used)
 • Interactional behaviors and role performances
 • Group norms, values, and behaviors

AS EXPRESSED IN VARIED DOMAINS OF DAILY LIVING

Source: Valle, 1990a.

Figure 2.3 Cultural assessment working model.

CULTURAL MAPPING–ACCULTURATION CONTINUUM OUTLINE

In the dementing illness arena, the different concepts about culture are most often realized by the practitioner when he or she is making assessments of ethnically diverse individuals and family groups and working out specific care plans. The formulation of the acculturation continuum (Figure 2.1), as well as of the factors that can distort the cultural assessment (Figures 2.2 and 2.3), provide a blueprint for the

cultural mapping discussion throughout the remainder of Part One. In operational-
izing the proposed frameworks the professional or provider takes the following steps:

1. **The target ethnic group is placed within a historical context relative to
   its present locale.** An overall profile of the different members is drawn
   within this background information. Throughout this process the expectation
   is that the practitioner remains aware that the profile is very much in the
   form of a living history of the target ethnically diverse group members. This
   living history provides access to the dementia-affected person's life experience along with an assessment of past capabilities and interests that may
   have a bearing on the careplan that is developed. Generalities about the ethnic group as a whole are relevant only to the extent that the information is
   pertinent to the group members being served within the planned dementia-
   care intervention.

2. **The key language–communicational format preferences of the ethnic
   group members are identified and included within the cultural mapping–acculturation continuum profile being developed.** If the intercultural engagement undertaking is to go forward, a linguistic–communicational
   rapprochement must be initiated early in the process.

3. **The target ethnic group members' preferred interactional and relational customs and expectations are documented, especially in regard
   to help-seeking and help-accepting attitudes and behaviors and incorporated into the careplan.** Similarly, the customary practices and relational
   patterns of the ethnic group must be included within any proposed planned
   intercultural engagement effort that is undertaken.

4. **The target ethnic group's normative expectations, along with the members'
   value–belief orientations, are to be identified.** Special attention is paid to
   how the family members perceive the whole arena of dementing illness.
   Because the ethnic group will be encountered residing within the overall
   context of a host society, the practitioner can expect the ethnic group members' values and expectations to range throughout the acculturation continuum.
   This is to say, some group members will be more traditionally oriented relative to their culture-of-origin, whereas others will definitely be more acculturated, with still others found in the in-between, bicultural mode. However,
   with regard to dementing illness, many of the group members, including
   those who may be more acculturated, can be expected to have incomplete,
   and even more traditional, or *folk understandings* about dementia. For example, some may hold to the folk understanding about various conditions
   being a normal part of aging. To the extent that traditional orientations are
   present, the practitioner will need to extend culturally compatible connections between the proposed careplan and where the ethnically diverse group
   members may be with regard to their outlooks.

5. **Social status, socioeconomic, and literacy considerations related to the
   target ethnic group members are charted and appropriately distinguished from the cultural information being assembled.** As has been

indicated, however, these factors do have a bearing on a full understanding of the target ethnically diverse client group's functioning and are to be taken into account within the overall ethnic family group profile that is developed.

6. **All of the preceding assessments are combined with other information within the overall evaluative processes that are being conducted relative to a suspected underlying dementing illness.** In practice, the cultural mapping process, which includes a working understanding of the acculturation continuum as an analytical technique, is both an information-gathering activity and an interactional undertaking. When the process is completed it considerably reduces the amount of confusion and misinformation, or misunderstandings, that often present in the evaluation of ethnically diverse group members (Hinkle & Wolff, 1957; Jecker et al., 1995; Paniagua, 1994). Moreover, the approach allows the practitioner to relate to both the underlying illness affecting a specific ethnoculturally diverse elder and to the coping practices of the client's family/significant others.

END NOTE: WHAT DOES CULTURE DO? A BRIEF REVIEW

In keeping with the central theme of the discussion here, it is important for the professional and provider to keep in mind that culture covers all of the facets of interpersonal relations. It assists individuals and groups not only to make sense of what is going on in their lives but to also cope with events such as a family member's affliction with a dementing illness. Culture also influences one's future actions. This is to say that individuals and groups act on the basis of patterns of values and customs that they have acquired and developed over time. This is not to deny that individuals make personal value and belief accommodations within their lives; however, families and the ethnic groups often act against the backdrop of their specific linguistic and value–belief systems. Moreover, these actions occur regardless of whether the individual, family, or ethnic group as a whole gives conscious attention to their beliefs and values. With these considerations in mind, culture can be said to perform the following functions:

- it filters how a message is heard and interpreted,
- it conditions how a person responds to the message,
- it plays a role in help-seeking and help-accepting communications and behaviors,
- it influences individual and group attitudes and actions,
- it influences future actions.

Chapter 3

Acquiring an Intercultural Knowledge Base

APPROACHING THE TASK

Given the trends in ethnic diversity delineated in Chapter 1, it is evident that inter-action with other cultures has become a very common aspect of modern life. However, this interaction does not automatically lead to understanding. Therefore, to establish intercultural proficiency, the professionals and providers working in the arena of dementing illness must take intercultural contact to higher levels by actively acquiring a cross-cultural knowledge base (Brislin, 1993; Brownlee, 1978; Cushner & Brislin, 1996; Gudykunst, 1994; Ivey, 1994; Ridley & Lingle, 1996; Teri et al., 1992; Triandis et al., 1990). Generally, the practitioners will find their service catchment area to be ethnically complex. Most dementia-service organizations include many different ethnic groups within their service boundaries. In fact, the professional or the provider cannot always know in advance who will be coming for services. Anyone from any ethnic group within the multicultural environment could appear at the service organization's doorstep. At the same time clients will come to the agency with their own unique ethnic orientations and understandings about dementing illness. Moreover, they will come with their own languages and will have cultural expecta-tions about how the service exchange is to be conducted.

The solution to the problem of the complex service environment is that the pro-fessional or provider retain a readiness to proceed from both a multicultural and ethnic-specific perspective. Practitioners must not only maintain a general alertness to multicultural diversity but they must also develop a strong knowledge base directly applicable to the ethnic group being targeted for services (Young et al., 1996). In implementing this dual approach the practitioner takes several practical steps to acquire a cross-cultural perspective (Song & Kim, 1993; Stewart, 1972). Specifically, these include: (a) developing a detailed awareness of the multicultural dimensions of the social environment, (b) making ethnic-specific knowledge connections by studying the ethnocultural group being targeted for services, (c) gaining an understanding of the current historical profile of the ethnic group being targeted, and (d) reconnecting all of the information gathered to the context of the multicultural environment (Brownlee, 1978; Valle, 1980b). Admittedly, the development of comprehensive intercultural capabilities requires the investment of time and effort in the strategy. There are practical limits, such as how far the knowledge development effort should actually be extended. The way to obviate practical difficulties that can arise is to make sure that the information search tasks are well planned out. Such planning can be handled in much the same manner as other kinds of professional skills development processes are undertaken. Therefore, the assumption is that the task will be approached systematically and that the information search effort will be broken down into manageable time-and-effort units. This will make the acquisition of both multicultural and ethnic-specific, dementia-focused knowledge a realistic achievement. There are a variety of reliable guides to community study that can be readily adapted to the ethnic group knowledge development task. For example, one can undertake the task from a community-study perspective, which has a tradition in the literature that extends back over several decades (Kinneman, 1947; Suttles, 1972; Vidich, Bensman, & Stein, 1964; Warren, 1955, 1973) and continues through to the present (Fellin, 1995; Hardcastle et al., 1997; Rivera & Erlich, 1992). The effort can also be approached from a field research perspective (Loftland & Loftland, 1995; Schatzman & Strauss, 1973). Collectively, these and other similar resources can direct the practitioner to a variety of productive ways to view the community. The strategies include ways to document the diversity of people and their needs, as well as the organizational processes and arrangements present within one's service environment. From an ethnocultural standpoint, the community-study strategies are quite adaptable to tracking the cultural–historical presence of groups within one's service catchment. Without the investment in community awareness, practitioners and their parent service organizations stand the chance of remaining quite isolated from their ethnically diverse work environment. They will be neither ready to target specific ethnic groups for services nor prepared for the eventual variety of ethnic groups asking for assistance.

MULTICULTURAL AWARENESS AS A STARTING POINT

The gaining of multicultural awareness is a starting point for the development of an intercultural knowledge base. Becoming multiculturally aware applies equally to practitioners who are bicultural as well as those who are strictly monocultural English-speakers coming from the mainstream U.S. host society. As has been noted, being bicultural may give the practitioner an edge in understanding the multicultural social environment. However, biculturality does not automatically make the professional or practitioner multicultural. Biculturality can certainly predispose the practitioner to work across many cultures. However, *ethnocentrism*—focusing one's perceptions only on the cultures that one knows—remains a very powerful force. Ethnocentrism can inhibit even the bicultural practitioner from reaching out to multiple cultures if the preparatory conceptual work is not done. Another inhibitor is when practitioners are not comfortable with their biculturality, that is, the professional or provider has not resolved the inner tensions and ambiguities that can accompany the simultaneous "straddling" of two different cultures. Therefore, a caveat must be stated when indicating that being bicultural "may give the practitioner an edge" in the multicultural engagement arena. In such instances, professionals or practitioners must have worked through their inner doubts and tendency toward their own type of ethnocentrism and come to a conscious sense of direction in moving across multiple cultural formats. As indicated earlier, the United States has been, and remains, a multiethnic society (Bahr, Chadwick, & Stauss, 1979; Greer, 1974; Hraba, 1994; Pedraza & Rumbaut, 1996; Rogers, 1996). If one looks at the social environment closely one can see that, even in the country's most isolated areas, ethnic diversity persists. The United States has been diverse from its origins. In what became the 13 colonies, settlers gradually grew ethnically apart from their homelands. Diversity was present even among the country's original people, the Native Americans/American Indians. There were different tribes, customs, and language systems among the Native Americans, just as there are today (Trimble et al., 1996). This diversity has accelerated throughout the continuing 400-year history of the United States as wave after wave of immigrants landed on the nation's shores and as vast territories were obtained through purchase or conquest (McLemore, 1994). The Louisiana Purchase of 1803 added the whole area of what is now the heartland, or midwestern part of the country. The treaty of Guadalupe–Hidalgo in 1848, at the end of the war with Mexico, added what are large sections of the western and southwestern United States. The conclusion of the Spanish–American War in 1898 brought with it many offshore territories, such as Puerto Rico and other islands of the Caribbean, along with U.S. Guam. In each of these and other instances, it was not just land that was acquired, but different peoples, with their unique languages and customs of their homelands of origin. Recognition of the country's multiethnicity, whether acknowledged or not by the mainstream society, must nonetheless be consciously recognized by the professional and provider working in the dementing illness arena.

As a second step, the practitioner must look outward to the community as a whole to determine which ethnic groups are represented within the designated service region. Because the focus of this text is on late onset dementing illness, many questions can be asked at this stage. What are the relative sizes of the different ethnic groups? What are the proportions of elderly within the ranks of the different ethnic groups that are found? What are the service use patterns of the different ethnocultural populations in general? Have the members of any of the various ethnic groups been coming forward seeking dementia-related services? If so, what are the specific caregiving needs that have been expressed? The answers to these questions can assist the professional or provider to develop a working plan for engaging the different sectors of the multicultural community. Moreover, specific ethnic groups to be targeted for services can be better identified in this way and, their needs can be prioritized.

In the third step toward developing multicultural readiness, the professional or provider moves to the practical action. Actual information gathering is undertaken with respect to the ethnic populations that are encountered, and service planning efforts are completed, to include sequencing the ethnic groups to be targeted given practitioner and parent organization resources in terms of time and personnel.

As noted in the Preface, an easy initial action to gain an overview of the ethnic diversity in one's own community is to browse through the local telephone directories. The notations about ethnic restaurants, churches, self-help associations, and community-service organizations, along with the surname listings of individuals, can provide a powerful impression about the underlying multiethnic configuration of one's community.

Driving or taking public transportation through different communities in one's service region can likewise enhance an awareness of local ethnic diversity. Billboards and storefront signs in other languages can reinforce the impression obtained. In fact, these actions are suggested as an important part of either a self-directed or an agency-sponsored multicultural training exercise and blend well with the "analyzing social settings" approach suggested by Schatzman and Strauss (1973) and Loftland and Loftland (1995).

From a more formal perspective, the practitioner can turn to health and human service directories. These are available in most regions and are used to support information and referral activity. Here the practitioner can find listings not only of mainstream services but also of ethnically focused programs. As part of the multicultural effort, calls and visits can be undertaken to selected settings that serve ethnically diverse populations. In this manner the professional or provider can get to know the community first hand. Also, in return, the organizations serving specific ethnic populations can get to know more about dementing illness and other available resources.

In addition, the practitioner can access a variety of planning documents available within the service catchment area. Examples include the long-range plans of the Area Agencies on Aging, the United Way, and local public health departments. This is to name but three types of readily available regionally focused documents that collectively can provide overviews of the region's ethnic diversity. Often these kinds of documents contain individualized demographic profiles of specific communities within the overall service region, along with projections of the needs for the area's population groups. From a broader perspective, the practitioner can turn to the U.S. censuses and various interpretive documents that emerge within a few years after the last census. The practitioner can also turn to various data centers within one's own state or county, or regional planning groups, to obtain additional overviews of the different populations residing within one's catchment area.

Professionals or providers should not limit themselves to the types of area-planning documents just mentioned. Rather, practitioners should explore other reports that may be available from local public and private organizations, including many groups that are not formally chartered but that meet regularly to exchange information and coordinate services within designated locales. Often these provider councils focus on specific problems or kinds of programs, such as long-term care services. Many times these groups develop background papers about the populations serviced as well as local problems. Moreover, at times they include information about ethnic group needs that perhaps are not found in other documents. It is difficult to name the documents and organizations for every region in the United States, because each locale has developed its own multicultural information. It is certain, however, that some pertinent information is available for the gathering. One needs only make a decided effort to seek it out.

What may be disappointing for the professional or provider specializing in dementia care is how little information there may be related to dementing illness with regard to ethnically diverse populations, especially related to the professional or provider's particular regions. This condition will vary from region to region, although in some areas, because of local interest in dementing illness and ethnicity, there can at times be surprisingly relevant findings. This may occur where there are active Alzheimer's disease–focused service and research organizations that have taken the multicultural message to heart. However, the overall picture with regard to dementing illness among ethnically diverse populations looks to remain quite uneven, varying from region to region, for several years to come. What often seems to happen is that both the formal service sector and the local ethnic community service infrastructure agencies focus on problems that appear more pressing to them than dementing illness.

Therefore, it will most likely be up to the individual practitioners to shape the profile of dementing illness among ethnically diverse groups within their local region. However, despite this and other difficulties noted, the central value of undertaking the development of the multicultural profile will be in having professionals and providers familiarize themselves with the true ethnic diversity of their service communities. Moreover, professionals and providers can be spurred on to more intensive work by the firsthand knowledge of the groups in need with regard to Alzheimer's disease and dementing illnesses. As will be discussed in subsequent chapters, ethnically diverse peoples may give different names and meanings to the signs and symptoms of dementing illness, but to date no cultural group in the United States with an elderly cohort has appeared to escape the ravages of dementing illness processes.

The underlying principle for both the professional or provider as well as the parent service organization is to be alert to linguistic and cultural variety among the client ethnic groups that require dementia-related services. Therefore, before rushing to serve only one ethnic group, practitioners and their parent service organizations must recognize the heterogeneity of the whole social environment. From this stronger planning position the organization and the professional or provider can proceed to ethnic-specific service targeting.

It may be true that because of existing in-house bilingual/bicultural resources, and already established linkages, a specific ethnic group (or groups) will be scheduled for immediate contact. Nonetheless, practitioners and their parent service organizations must be able to respond to inquiries by ethnically diverse family members not enrolled in their current service programs. Over a period of time, the professional or provider will find that word-of-mouth communications carry across from ethnic group to ethnic group. A successful program conducted with one ethnic population in the dementing illness arena has the potential for cross-cultural impact on others. Eventually multiple ethnic groups will seek help. For these reasons a proactive multicultural engagement readiness needs to be maintained.

ETHNIC-SPECIFIC CONNECTION

From the stage of multi-ethnic/multicultural awareness, the professional and provider is ready to make ethnic-specific connections. Taking the initial step of becoming multiculturally knowledgeable enables the practitioner to be more effective about making ethnic-specific targeting and resource mobilization decisions. The social environment may be diverse, but ethnic groups are unique. Each group presents its own language and customs and has its own closely held beliefs and normative expectations. These unique patterns need to be taken into account when planning interventions and implementing dementia-related programs. In terms of effective intercultural work, the professional or provider must approach dementia-affected elders and their caregivers on an individualized, one-ethnic-group-at-a-time basis. This is not to negate the fact that the multiculturally capable practitioner may have ongoing responsibilities for diverse clients from different ethnic groups. This circumstance can be a fact of life for many professionals or providers. Rather, the issue at stake is that the practitioner avoid inappropriate cultural generalizations and focus on the needs of the target ethnic group members. For example, many traditionally oriented ethnocultural groups favor family- or group-oriented intervention approaches. In some cultures the family or group may be more patriarchally oriented; in others there may be a more matriarchal-type decision system. In some cultures very distant kin are part of the immediate network; others may have more nuclear type formats, even though this "nucleus" is actually an extended, multigenerational family cluster rather than what the literature views as the nuclear family of the parents and the children.

To make the ethnic-specific connection the professional or provider proceeds in a systematic manner to specifically understand the target ethnic group's historical presence within the social environment as well as its current status. In so doing, the professional or provider applies a *cultural-search* orientation to the more classic problem-solving approach, adding a dementing illness perspective. The generic problem-solving method includes problem assessment, development of an intervention plan or strategy, an intervention, and evaluation of the overall effort. In the culture search approach the professional or provider:

1. assesses the ethnic client group's situation with reference to dementia-specific concerns in the context of the group member's cultural orientations and understandings,
2. develops a service plan blending the dementia related needs and the ethnic client group's cultural response patterns,
3. implements the plan in the light of what has been discovered/what is known about the ethnic groups cultural history and present coping approaches, and
4. evaluates and modifies the overall effort with a dementia focus, and also with a definite eye to the cultural underpinnings of the situation.

The assumption is that the professional or provider will be familiar with a problem-solving methodology, in whatever way it is formulated within particular disciplines. As indicated in Chapter 1, a further assumption is made that the practitioner is knowledgeable about dementing illness. However, the interculturally competent practitioner also incorporates the cultural elements of language preferences, the group's cultural expectations about rapport and trust, its decision-making style, and its underlying values and beliefs into the problem-solving process.

UNDERSTANDING THE GROUP'S HISTORICAL PRESENCE

If a choice has to be made about where to begin, the focus should be on the ethnic group's history—not just its general cultural history, but rather the group's immediate past and current history within the practitioner's service region. In starting the process, the practitioner must be aware that each ethnic group has a number of key historical indicators that can yield a composite cultural profile of ethnic family life and its individual members. These indicators include:

- a historical past that takes into account the ethnic group member's country-of-origin from which the group's long-standing traditions are derived; a historical presence within the host society of the United States; this includes the overall group's and the individual family's time and place of entry to the United States, along with whether the entry was voluntary and desired or forced by circumstances in the home country;
- a very unique local history in the community where the ethnic group members now reside; and
- a variety of individual or personal accommodations that have been made within the context of acculturation influence; here the practitioner looks to how the ethnic group members engage the host society in different aspects of their lives, such as in the workplace, in the service setting where the family may be coming for assistance with the dementing illness concerns, and at home.

A fairly concise overview of the target ethnic group can be constructed by walking through the various steps as just outlined. For example, knowledge about the target ethnic group's culture of origin can furnish an important backdrop of the meaning of traditions and customs that are encountered. Awareness of the ethnic group's history in the United States can provide insight on the group member's accommodations to the effects of modernization and shifts from the country-of-origin orientations. For example, does the group still rely on its own traditional medical practices? If so, then who are some of the indigenous practitioners who can be incorporated as allies into the proposed dementia-focused intervention plan? Are there other cultural customs that can be, or need to be, included as well (Paniagua, 1994)?

Attention to the ethnic group's presence in the local environment can assist the professional or provider to recognize possible barriers to the service linkage component of the intervention plan that will be proposed. For instance, is there a local track record among agencies for assisting members of the target ethnic group with services other than dementia-related programming? Finally, attention to the individual and family group responses with reference to both their own cultural history and to their adjustment to the host U.S. cultural society will enable the practitioner to individualize the interventions that are proposed. Here, the acculturation continuum formulation discussed in Chapter 2 can be made especially applicable. Some of the client ethnic group members will be found at the more traditional side of the continuum. This will most likely include the dementia-affected elder and the primary caregiver. Other family members will be found to be mostly at the acculturated side of the continuum. Still others will be bicultural, straddling both the traditional and mainstream cultures.

The only way that this vital information can be obtained is to take the historical pulse of the target ethnic group in some systematic fashion. In actual practice, the above approach is not linear. Professionals and providers will often find themselves moving back and forth from content about individuals to information about the group as a whole. The issue is not to get stuck slavishly following an outline but rather to eventually conduct an evaluation that satisfies all of the points suggested throughout the assessment process.

It is understood that it is not always easy to proceed in the manner outlined. In fact, to the beginner the undertaking may appear quite formidable and time consuming. In the context of present caseloads, how much more effort can be asked of individual practitioners? In addition, from the dementia-service organization point of view, the cultural history information-gathering activity may be seen as incongruent with the cost-containment norms that pervade the service sector. At the same time, a sense of balance must be inserted into the approach to be taken. In some respects everyone is a beginner at some time, or at some place in one's practice. Normal professional caution should not be interpreted as a rationale for inaction.

Moreover, if sincere goodwill is extended by the professional or provider, the information-gathering–background-knowledge development task is able to be encompassed within one's workload, and it is even a pleasant undertaking. Regardless of whether one is a beginner or a seasoned practitioner, people who are knowledgeable about the target ethnic group, who are able to assist in the learning effort, can be found. From an overall perspective, this ethnic history–ethnic familiarization activity on the part of the professional or provider has a big payoff for all concerned. For example, ethnic group members with traditional culture-of-origin understandings about dementing conditions, and about Alzheimer's disease in particular, may not have incorporated what is currently known about these conditions from a medical and scientific perspective. By being aware of this, the practitioner can build appropriate informational bridges, saving potential hours of misunderstandings.

Moreover, cultural-familiarizing efforts on the part of the professional or provider can also be an important means of identifying key concerns the ethnic group members may have about relating to formal service systems. This familiarization effort is also an excellent means to connect with the group's local norms (Cheng, 1987). The usual intake evaluation information for dementing illness, which often bypasses the in-depth cultural side of individual and family life, can be placed into a more comprehensive and relevant framework. For example, without such information, it could take much longer to decipher why the family members may be resisting the treatment plan.

The information may also reveal that the family members are upset with the apparent lack of a culturally attuned response from the practitioner or the practitioner's parent organization.

Cultural–historical background information will also facilitate a more relevant connection to the dementia-affected ethnic elder's immediate caregiving environment. For example, if Latinos are being targeted the professional or provider must know which Latino/Hispanic subgroup is being addressed. Despite a relatively common language base, Latinos/Hispanics are quite heterogeneous depending on their nationality-of-origin, as well as their time of entry into the United States and the conditions under which they entered. It is equally important to know if the ethnic group members are political or economic refugees. If elders are the original family pioneers to the United States, or if they are following their children who came earlier and are now being reunified through provisions of immigration policy, this will likewise make a difference. The pioneer elders will have come to the United States in a different era. They will have been exposed longer to the host society, and they will remember a culture-of-origin that may be different from how the culture of their homeland has evolved in the intervening years. The new elderly arrivals may be faced with many adjustments and culture shock experiences.

The same differentiations need to be applied with even greater meaning to other generically labeled ethnic groups, such as those considered within the broad category of Asian Americans. Here the professional or provider must drop the more global ethnic designation and focus on specific ethnocultural groups. For example, if the practitioner were to begin work with a dementia-affected Vietnamese elder it would be of importance to know if the family belongs to the first large wave of arrivals in 1975, or if they lived in the United States before that era, or if they came much later, as "boat people" (Owan, Bliatout, Lin, Liu, Nguyen, & Wong, 1985). Each family circumstance may bring different sets of coping resources to bear on the dementing illness. Each background profile may provide different sets of intercultural bridges from the Vietnamese culture to formal services. Each will impart unique cultural information to influence the overall assessment being made.

The same approach can be applied with reference to generational differences within still other ethnic cohorts. For example, if the professional or provider is targeting Japanese Americans, it is important to know if the dementia-affected elder is an *issei* (a first-generation arrival), a *nisei* (of the second generation—most likely from the World War II generation) or a *sansei* or *yansei* (of the third or fourth generation), although the practitioner will expect that the latter two groups will constitute the family members rather than the dementia-affected elders themselves. In the near future, there may be a sufficient large age 65+ *sansei* generation in the United States to begin to experience late-onset dementing illness.

The value of this information may emerge in interventions that will be able to link to specific reference points in the elder's long term memory. The importance of the particular background information will also show when the practitioner mobilizes the family's help-seeking and help-accepting orientations. A Japanese American *nisei* with dementing illness who lived in the United States at the outbreak of World War II may be reliving quite a different experience than a counterpart *nisei* who lived in

Japan during the same era. The Japanese American who lived in the United States would have most likely have experienced that period in 1943 when 110,000 Japanese Americans on the West coast were summarily uprooted from their homes and, within a 2-week period, found themselves confined to concentration camps with barbed wire and armed guards watching their every move (McLemore, 1994). In contrast a Japanese American *nisei* may be re-experiencing the events of a youth spent in Japan. As the dementing illness deepens, this individual might retain little memory of the U.S. part of her or his life experience.

Putting emphasis on understanding the historical presence of the ethnic group members stops the formation of inappropriate stereotypes. In addition, as professionals or providers become familiar with the historical context of ethnic groups they will likely be able to pinpoint the distinct experiences of the different-generation family members even within a single family. For example, knowing the experiences of the extended family group members at different times in the host society helps to identify important variations in outlooks of the various significant others and greatly assists in shaping of the service plan itself.

Similar approaches with different questions could be directed toward long-established groups within the U.S. ambience, such as African Americans, American Indians/Native Americans, and a host of other ethnic groups. The professional or provider will soon find how useful it is to know and understand differential experiences of ethnocultural groups in ethnic-specific terms.

It is important to know that the ethnic-specific historical–cultural information-gathering effort does not always involve extensive library searches, although written sources are a good place to start if one needs to become acquainted with the customs, beliefs, and cultural attitudes, as well as the socioeconomic and other status features, of the targeted ethnic group. There are a number of alternative information sources that can be tapped. Some of these potential sources have already been mentioned, such as the reports and long-range planning statements of various federal, state, and local organizations within the professional's or provider's service environment. Alternative sources include community events calendars, which now often appear in various media. There are usually any number of ethnic group events open to the general public that allow cultural outsiders to learn much about a specific ethnic group. One need not be Chinese to appreciate the significance of the Chinese New Year and engage in a part of the celebration.

There are also key informants, sometimes referred to as *cultural brokers* (to be discussed in depth in Chapter 11), who are knowledgeable about the ethnic community being targeted for services. These individuals can be invited to assist by providing important local information. Many of these key informants have worked and lived in the local community and can provide the kind of personal detail not found in reports and planning documents. These key informants/brokers can possibly be found throughout the infrastructure of community-based organizations serving the target ethnic community. They can also be found in the ethnic group's religious organizations, and even its business associations, neighborhood clubs, and Veterans Administration and affiliates, to mention but a few. It is important not to expect these brokers or informants to be knowledgeable about dementing illnesses—some might, but most will not. As their role will be outlined in the discussion in Chapter 11, suffice it to say here that links to the community key informants/brokers will decidedly help professionals and providers gain insight into the help-seeking and help-accepting beliefs and practices of the ethnic community.

All of the activity discussed is not intended to be simply a fact-gathering exercise. In addition to its use for careplanning for the family targeted for services, the information, once gathered, has lasting value. The broad outlines of the local history of the target ethnic group has a cumulative usefulness for application to other families from the same ethnic group coming for dementia-related assistance. In sum, the effort helps to shape the overall cultural mapping process.

BEING ABLE TO THINK MULTICULTURALLY AGAIN

Certainly, awareness of ethnic group differences, elaborated within ethnic-specific careplans, is a cornerstone of effective intercultural practice. Likewise, this practice is grounded in the awareness of individual differences in clients and the keeping of a watchful eye focused on the target ethnic group's history. With this said, however, the professional or provider must again be able to think in a multicultural manner. As noted earlier, the social environment surrounding most service organizations is quite ethnically heterogeneous. Therefore, it is incumbent on practitioners and their parent organizations to be able to engage their service worlds from a multicultural perspective also. Moreover, the social environment changes, as do service priorities. Over time, new ethnic group concentrations come into one's service region. The practitioner, as well as the organization, has to be ready to respond to the requests for services by the new arrivals. The future for the dementia-service arena is that of continued and growing diversity. It is at this juncture that practitioners and their parent service organizations need to be able to call on both their multicultural as well as their culture-specific capabilities.

DEVELOPING THE CULTURAL KNOWLEDGE BASE:
A REVIEW

To initiate the social mapping process, the professional or provider must acquire a solid knowledge base relative to both the overall ethnic diversity of the service environment and the specific ethnic group(s) being designated for services. A summary of several steps in the process includes the following considerations.

1. **The initial step for the professional or provider is to become multiculturally aware and knowledgeable.** This requires the practitioner to purposely examine the service environment and systematically catalog its diversity. Every item of information does not have to be written down, but key findings should be recorded. This task of documentation can be aided by the availability of both agency and personal computers, which permit for the easy insertions of corrections and updating of information.
2. **The type of multi-ethnic community scanning effort being suggested here**

can best be done effectively through an organized planning effort on the part of the professional or provider. The practitioner must proceed proactively rather than wait opportunistically to see which ethnic group will come forward with requests for help. This latter approach puts the practitioner and the parent organization in a continual catch-up position. Therefore, professionals and providers must prioritize the time and effort to be expended in undertaking the cultural and historical information search activity. They also need to make a realistic assessment of their own capabilities and those of their parent organizations to use the information gathered. Finally, the proactive knowledge development stance includes periodic examination of the cultural–historical information gathered, with appropriate updating.

3.   **To be most effective, the cultural–historical information search effort must be tailored for use with specific ethnic group(s).** As has been noted, the reality facing the practitioner at the point of service delivery is the need to be able to communicate meaningfully with the more monolingual members of specific ethnic groups. Therefore, although a balanced multicultural knowledge-gathering approach is suggested, the actual direct contact will be ethnic specific in nature. Eventually the information will need to be further tailored for application to specific family groups.

4.   **It is equally important that the professional and provider alike keep themselves focused on dementing illness,** although much of the available information on ethnically diverse populations may center around issues and concerns not directly related to dementing illness. There is an emerging body of work around dementing illness and specific ethnic groups. Sample sources are grouped below. The listings should not be considered as exhaustive but rather as providing a starting point for linking dementing illness knowledge as well as other related health and service concerns and issues to different ethnically diverse populations.

AFRICAN AMERICANS. With regard to African Americans the professional or provider can turn to Baker (1988), Barressi and Mennon (1990), Burton et al. (1995), Cox (1993), Dungee-Anderson and Beckett (1992), Fredman et al. (1995), Gaines (1988–1989), Haley et al. (1995), Heyman et al. (1991), Hinrichen and Ramirez (1992), Lawton et al. (1992), Lewis and Chavis Ausbery (1996), Mintzer and Macera (1992), Morycz et al. (1987), Mui and Burnette (1994), Schoenberg, Anderson, and Haerer (1985), Segal and Wykle (1988–1989), Wershow (1976), Wood and Parham (1990), Wykle and Segal (1991), and Young and Kahana (1995). An advantage of much of this literature is that it is comparative in nature, usually examining African Americans and Anglo populations.

AMERICAN INDIANS/NATIVE AMERICANS. When focusing on ethnically diverse groups from these populations, the practitioner can examine Cross (1996), Hendrie et. al. (1993), Hennessy and John (1995), Kramer (1991, 1992a, 1992b, 1996), Manson (1989, 1993), McDonald-Shoemaker (1981), Novak (1974), and Strong (1984).

ASIAN AMERICANS/PACIFIC ISLANDERS. Content on ethnic groups

from this ethnically diverse population group encompasses a range of ethnic subgroups, including Chamorros (Fegurgur, 1995; Haddock & Santos, 1992; Lavine et al., 1991; Zhang et al., 1990), Chinese (Chu, 1991; Katzman et al., 1988; Liu, Lin, et al., 1991; Liu, Tsou, et al., 1991; Serby et al., 1987), and Japanese (Elliot et al., 1996; Homma et al., 1994; Kobayashi et al., 1993; Nakano, 1991; Tempo & Saito, 1996).

LATINOS/HISPANICS. In looking to Latino/Hispanic populations, the practitioner can examine Arámbula (1992); Aranda (1987); Burns (1992); Cox and Monk (1993); Eribes and Bradley-Rawls (1978); Gallagher-Thompson, Talamantes, Ramirez, and Valverde (1996); Henderson and Gutierrez-Mayka (1992); Mintzer et al. (1992); Mintzer, Rupert, & Herman (in press); Pi et al. (1996); Purdy and Arguello (1992); Siddarthan and Sowers-Hoag (1989); Sizemore et al. (1991); Talamantes et al. (1996); Valle (1994); and Yaniz (1990). Also, Cox and Monk (1990) examine African Americans and Hispanics and compare these two ethnic groups with Anglos (Cox & Monk, 1993), and Henderson et al. (1993) report on African Americans and Hispanics.

MIXED ETHNIC GROUPS/OVERARCHING ISSUES OF DEMENTIA AMONG ETHNICALLY DIVERSE POPULATIONS. The practitioner can access Advisory Panel on Alzheimer's Disease (1993); Alzheimer's Disease and Related Disorders Association (1994); Aranda & Knight (1997); "Culture and Caregiving" (1992); Henderson (1987, 1990a, 1990b); Henderson and Gutierrez-Mayka (1992); Lilienfeld and Perl (1994); Lockery (1987, 1991); Mintzer (1994); Mintzer, Macera, et al. (in press); Morrison (1982); Ng (1994); Ogunniyi and Osuntokun (1991); Osuntokun, Ogunniyi, Lekwauwa, Norton, and Pillay (1992); Rossenthal (1986); Saldov and Chow (1994); Schrafft (1980); Tallmer, Mayer, and Hill (1977); Valle (1981, 1988–1989, 1990a, 1992b); Valle et al. (1989, 1994); and Yeo and Gallagher-Thompson (1996).

In the absence of dementia-related content, the practitioner can make use of information from related areas, such as ethnic group member approaches to the care of frail elderly or of chronically ill patients regardless of the type of illness or age (Thomas & Rose, 1991). Regardless of the source of the problems being addressed, the practitioner may be able to glean cultural content for possible application to the dementia-care arena. The issue at hand is that the practitioner cannot always wait around for the necessary information to materialize. The needs of ethnically diverse family have to be met at the point of contact (Paniagua, 1994).

A very possible side outcome of the professional's or provider's efforts to assemble whatever culturally relevant dementia-related information can be gathered is that, over time, the practitioners and/or their parent organizations will find themselves with a rich source of ethnic-specific dementia-care material. This content can then in turn be used for internal intercultural consumption, to include staff training and competency upgrading purposes as well as sharing of the information with other professionals and providers to enhance their work with dementia-affected ethnic group members.

5. **Throughout the cultural-historical knowledge building process, the professional and provider must guard against overgeneralizations and stereotyping.** No one ethnic or family group will incorporate all the aspects of what is discovered about their cultural roots. In addition, groups and individuals will change over time. Moreover, dementing illness brings its own set of stressors, which can modify even the most ingrained of cultural orientations. Therefore, although the cultural and historical information gathered may yield a number of general characteristics about the ethnic group and its traditions, the practitioner must be alert as to how these generalizations play out, one family, and one situation, at time. Seasoned practitioners may be able to set an example. There is no question that personal biases and stereotypes need to be addressed. As Gudykunst (1994) indicates, there is a strong tendency to operate out of fixed categories—or stereotypes—thereby setting boundaries on the knowledge about others and their culture. As Gudykunst (1994, p. 19) further indicates, there is a need to constantly extend the "width" of these categories. One way to do so is to use self-reflection, facing one's biases directly, expanding one's core information. Other avenues include staff and community feedback sessions in which ethnic-focused information is regularly enhanced and updated.

6. **In addition, in regard to the actual information-gathering aspect of the direct client assessment, the practitioner needs to consider documenting the client group's living arrangements (Himes, Hogan, & Eggebeen, 1996).** This includes not only the immediate living situation of the dementia-affected elder but also the overall neighborhood and broader community environment surrounding the client group. With regard to living arrangements, it is important to note that, in some families, the dementia-affected elder's care is rotated throughout the extended family. This practice can include the fact that the elder will live for selected months in different households, to include locations in another city, county, or state. Such careplans may fit the family's care values, but they may need periodic evaluation relative to the dementia-affected elder's progressive decline, which may bring added disorientation and the centralizing of care in one household.

Basically, then, the two parts of the intercultural knowledge development activity, namely, to focus on the ethnic-specific needs of the client group and the overall multicultural social environment, work in a complementary fashion. This dual focus can address the direct needs of the patient highlighted throughout Parts One and Two while at the same time facilitate the community outreach and networking aspects of the comprehensive cultural mapping approach highlighted in Chapter 13.

END NOTE

The overall process of developing both an ethnic-specific and a multicultural information base on dementia serves as the cornerstone of the cultural mapping process. The allocation of time and effort to this aspect of the overall cultural mapping task has long-term yield with reference to providing a strong foundation for intercultural understanding. The outcomes of developing the knowledge base and the cultural–historical profile of the ethnic group or groups being targeted for dementia-care services can be made applicable throughout the ongoing process of intercultural contact with the client families.

Chapter 4

Language: A Key Point of Cultural Contact

Just as language is a point of entry to another culture, so it is a line of demarcation between cultures. Language is the symbol system that provides an understanding of the underlying structure of how a group thinks and believes (Nunes, 1995). It has such importance that some observers put language and culture together in one term: *langaculture* (Agar, 1994). It is one thing to get to know a group through its documents and background history; it is quite another to engage the culture directly through its preferred channels of communication. Therefore, in entering the language and communication phase of the cultural mapping process, the professional and provider must be prepared to use the ethnic group's native idiom. Forcing English on monolingual ethnically diverse group members, or on those who prefer their native language, is not acceptable. This is especially so in light of the problems faced by the dementia-affected patient, who may have lost access to English as a second language (Ekman, Wahlin, Norberg, & Winblad, 1993).

Language access can take two routes. The first and obvious point of entry is that the practitioner would be bilingual with respect to the ethnic group being targeted for dementia-care services. Failing this, the second approach is to have the language entry capability available in a surrogate form, that is, the professional or provider would have competent bilingual communication assistance relative to the target ethnic client group. In this case, because the practitioner is not bilingual he or she would call on the parent dementia-care agency's bilingual personnel resource pool. Failing this, the professional or provider would then turn to the *bicultural communication pair* strategy. The bicultural-pair arrangement teams a monolingual English-speaking but dementia-capable practitioner with a bilingual/bicultural fellow practitioner (McDaniel, 1996). This individual can be a culturally and linguistically attuned consultant, or volunteer community person, or cultural broker from the target ethnic group.

The discussion below will expand on these roles as they are implemented within the cultural mapping process. In addition, the discussion will highlight a number of cultural mapping techniques related to engaging ethnically diverse clients on their own linguistic turf. These include: (a) avoiding the creation of conflicts of interest by depending on family members as the primary intercultural communicators (b) learning to build personal intercultural communicational capabilities through advance preparation and the judicious deployment of the bicultural-pair approach, and (c) developing a working understanding of the underlying principles of communication exchange theory in an intercultural context. In this regard the practitioner must remain alert to all aspects of the messages coming from or going to the ethnically diverse group members (Braun et al., 1995; Gerontological Society of America, 1991; Sizemore et al., 1991), including the nonverbal and more symbolic aspects of the communication process (Cheng, 1987). The issue at stake in the dementing illness arena is that the professional or provider must be able to convey meaningful information in the appropriate linguistic format, as opposed to using *literally translated* ideas. The latter terminology may be technically correct but far removed from communicating an understandable message (Anrow Sciences of Mandex, Inc., 1987).

AVOIDING COMMUNICATIONAL CONFLICTS OF INTEREST

The first step in the intercultural communication process is not to place bilingual ethnic group family members in a conflict-of-interest position. It can be expected that many ethnically diverse families will have one or more members who can act as communication brokers (Grosjean, 1982). These individuals can be a great asset and should not be excluded from the proposed dementia-focused communication and careplanning effort. On the contrary, any available bilingual family members and caregiving significant others are to be encouraged to take an active role within the differential diagnostic process and the eventual careplan or intervention strategy that emerges. However, because there is a shortage of competent bilingual personnel, family members or friends and neighbors are often "drafted" by practitioners or their parent organizations for the role of the principal bilingual communicator. This is to be avoided. Except as a last resort, family members and significant others should not be made the principal go-betweens in the situation. Moreover, if there is no other alternative, the professional or provider should move with trepidation. Being placed in the role of the principal bilingual communicator could put the family member directly into a conflict-of-interest position: On the one hand the bilingual family members will be trying to maintain their own and the family's interests, and on the other hand they will be accommodating the dictates of the practitioner.

Admittedly, there is a fine line here, as some family members can take on the role of go-between in a relatively objective manner. Moreover, there will also be some occasions, particularly around crises situations, when the monolingual English-speaking professional or provider will have no reasonable alternative but to ask for the interpretive help of a family member. However, even here the English-speaking practitioner must avoid the temptation of making the family bilingual go-between the mainstay of the intercultural communication exchange and dementia-care planning effort. There are several reasons for this caution. First, in most instances the mono-lingual English-speaking professional or provider will not be able to tell if undue pressure is being placed on the family go-between. Likewise, the practitioner will not be able to know with certainty if the key dementing illness messages are getting through to the ethnically diverse family members, as intended. Eventually, the astute practitioner will recognize that something is amiss, especially when carefully crafted careplans do get underway, but this insight can come much later in the overall dementia assessment and intervention process.

Second, in many instances the family member being placed in the pseudo-practi-tioner role may lack the necessary technical or health background relative to commu-nicating the more medical aspects of dementing illness. This places an extra burden on the bilingual family communicator who, like all the other family members, may be seeking relief rather than more work. Third, it can happen that the bilingual family member in the pseudo-professional role may indeed have an understanding about the technical side of dementing illness but, because of family dynamics, may not be in a position to impart the knowledge gained. Finally, in some cultures, status alone can block appropriate communication; for example, younger family members, or those with lower family status, may feel inhibited in discussing specific topics with the older, higher status family members (Elliot et al., 1996).

> Case 4.1. The López family requested a diagnostic evaluation of Mr. López's symptoms of blackouts, seizures, and some memory loss accompanied by behavioral problems. The outcome of the diagnosis was dementia of neurosyphilitic origin. The clinic had an overload of patients to process and an exit interview was scheduled at the earliest time convenient for the staff. Unfortunately, the clinic's only bilingual staff member was away on leave. As both the patient and Mrs. López were monolingual Spanish speakers, their daughter trans-lated at the exit interview. A week later Mrs. López phoned the bilingual staff member angrily complaining that her doctor called and said that she needed to come in to be tested for the presence of a venereal infection because of her husband's diagnosis. In the conver-sation it was clear that the daughter had been too embarrassed to discuss with her mother the sexually transmitted origins of her father's dementing condition and had translated the diagnosis as related to her father's lifelong explosive temperament as an *enojn* (a person given to irrational bouts of anger). The daughter had also not understood that the clinic physicians were required to report Mr. López diagnosis. The bilingual staff member ex-plained why her family physician had been notified and the importance of Mrs. López following up with the tests. She apologized for having been away, but indicated that she had been on a planned leave. She then set up a home visit date to go over a careplan.

It must be stated clearly that no argument is being raised against involving all of the family members, especially the more bilingual members, in the overall dementia assessment and careplan process. The issue at hand is simply not to overload these individuals by asking them to perform both the role of concerned family member and practitioner. Moreover, if the professionals or providers are not themselves bilingual and bicultural, they are faced with further difficulties by entering cultural territory while not understanding the target ethnic group's cultural protocols. In Case 4.1, above, the daughter did not consider it appropriate to discuss her father's sexual life and did not convey to her mother the importance that the mother herself be tested for the presence of a venereal infection. If dementia assessment and careplanning are truly to move into the bicultural/multicultural engagement arena, other arrangements will have to be made. In Case 4.1, postponement of the exit interview until the bilingual staff member could be present would have made a major difference in cultural understanding outcomes. Other alternatives could include hiring additional bilingual/bicultural staff, forming bicultural-pair arrangements, and instituting intercultural communication training programs within the dementia care organization. Any or all of these steps would have helped prevent the cultural shame and embarrassment in the López situation.

BUILDING INTERCULTURAL COMMUNICATIONAL READINESS

As a part of the overall intercultural communication preparation process, the professional or provider can take several steps. For bilingual practitioners, the task may be somewhat easier in that they potentially have built-in linguistic access to the target ethnic group. However, there may be some deceptively subtle barriers. For example, the bilingual practitioner may be rusty in the target ethnic group's language, not having used it for some time. It could also be that the practitioner may have learned the language in school in a nonconversational format. In such cases the bilingual professional or provider may be more at ease with the formal side of the native language rather than its colloquial counterpart. In other instances the practitioner may not be familiar with the local/regional modifications that have crept into the everyday discourse of the family members. Moreover, the ethnically diverse family members' capabilities may not extend to being able to handle technical terms even in their own native language. All of these obstacles will need to be considered and handled (Brownlee, 1978, pp. 68–78). The bilingual professional or provider has to be able to start the communicational exchange at the linguistic level where the family is found while at the same time remaining ready to infuse the complexities of dementing illness content appropriately into the conversation.

> Case 4.2. In trying to help the Latino Padilla family, the doctor had told the nurse to "tell the caregiver that Mrs. Padilla's *cognitive capabilities* are now severely impaired by the Alzheimer's disease type dementia." The message was translated literally to the caregiver and family members present as *Las capacitaciones cognoscitivos de su Mamá estan deterioradas.* The family members nodded politely to the bilingual professional but looked to one another without understanding. None of the adults present had education beyond the third grade. They had no idea what the concept of *capacitaciones conoscitivos* (cognitive capabilities) meant. At this point, the nurse realized what was going on and took another tack. She *transculturated* the message, saying, "The part of your mother's head that allows her to function like everyone else is damaged. It doesn't work anymore." This change of direction appeared to work. The family members began talking to each other and asked further questions.

In the everyday world of providing services to ethnically diverse groups, the bilingual/bicultural professional or provider will encounter complex communicational situations. This is true even when only one ethnic group is targeted for service. When different families within the ethnic group begin to interact with the practitioner, he or she has to be ready to deal with the many variations in linguistic and communicational preferences that arise (Grosjean, 1982). For example, in some instances the caregiving significant others, as well as the dementia-affected elder, may be completely monolingual, using only their native language. In other situations, some of the family caregivers may be bilingual, although this might not include the primary caregiver, with whom eventual face-to-face exchanges will have to be conducted.

In still other circumstances, the ethnic group members may use their native language at home but will attempt to communicate in English with people outside the home. However, the English used may be limited with respect to understanding of the more technical aspects of dementing illness as they are communicated to the family members. As a rule of thumb, however linguistically mixed the ensuing dialogue becomes, the bilingual/bicultural practitioner must be ready for all of the eventualities and be able to communicate appropriately with all of the key players in the caregiving situation.

In each of these instances it is vital that the professional or provider keep in mind that many ethnically diverse groups have not yet been exposed in depth to current medical and scientific information about Alzheimer's disease, or other dementing conditions for that matter. Therefore, the professional or provider must not only be able to assess the ethnic group members' language preferences and capabilities but must also be alert to their command of the technical elements of dementing disorders information that need to be communicated. In Case 4.2 the nurse recognized the fact that her statements about Mrs. Padilla's diagnosis were going over the heads of the family members. She quickly reversed to a more colloquial pattern of speech. The interculturally experienced communicator can also make such evaluations up front, usually in opening moments of the dialogue with ethnic group family members. The practitioner listens to the words that are used and the way the ideas are being framed. These early exchanges offer clues as to the ethnic client group's general level of language use, ranging from primarily using colloquial terminology through reliance on more technical and formal language usage. The Padilla family was obviously closer to the colloquial end of the spectrum of their native Spanish.

Advance Preparations

There are many ways to prepare for intercultural communication situations. In Chapter 1 the practitioner was advised about the necessity becoming knowledgeable about the *historical presence* of the ethnic group being targeted for services. Similarly, professionals and providers engaged in cultural mapping activities have to become alert to the *language presence* of the group members.

Generally speaking, the professional or provider can expect that the language of preference will emerge at the point of contact with the family members. At the same time, initial preparation is a must for the practitioner. For example, in more established dementia-service organizations, case records can be checked. Referral sources can likewise be contacted prior to the point of actual engagement with the family. Many times referring practitioners are quite knowledgeable about the family. An advance phone call to the family itself can also provide information about language preferences.

The Bicultural Communication Pair

It is recognized that not all service organizations will have sufficient bilingual/bicultural staff on board, especially with regard to the multiple ethnic groups to be found in many locales. This is why the concept of *bicultural-pairing* is suggested. Here, the English-speaking monocultural professional or provider links with a trained and experienced health or human services staff member, or a similarly equipped consultant, or a community person who is bilingual and bicultural with respect to the ethnic group being targeted for services. There are three expectations of the bicultural-pair candidates. First, the candidate selected as the "culturally compatible" member of the bicultural-pair must also be well versed in the target ethnic group members' language, including the colloquial formats being used locally. Second, each bilingual-pair candidate must also be attuned to the cultural value outlooks and expectations of the target ethnic group members. It is not enough to be linguistically in sync with the ethnically diverse clients. Rather, the individual selected for the cultural component of the bicultural-pair must be able also to provide insight into the ethnic group members' overall cultural orientations. Third, the bicultural-pair candidate must also be able to provide direct cross-cultural communication about dementing illness to the target ethnic group family members. In this regard, the bicultural member of the bicultural-pair has to keep watch on the family members' ability to understand the technical aspects of the Alzheimer's/dementia message and inform the monocultural English-speaking member of the team about the progress being made. Basically, the bicultural candidate becomes the cultural eyes and ears of the bicultural-pair arrangement.

Unfortunately, potential bicultural-pairs are not always available either in the numbers or at the times needed. Hence the practitioner must plan ahead to have the bilingual/bicultural resource person(s) available for the family session or contact. Once the bicultural-pair is formed, further advance preparations need to be made. This will include briefings in English and a review of the broad outlines of the planned home visit or office conference, along with the specifics of the Alzheimer's disease or other dementing condition information that will be discussed at the session. The professional or provider cannot assume in advance that the bicultural-pair candidate assisting in the communication will either know the specific case or be informed about dementing illness. At all costs, except perhaps when emergencies preclude advance preparation, the bicultural-pair team should not go into a situation "cold," especially at the beginning, when they are less experienced in working together, because the initial sessions can be linguistically exhausting. After some time, the ability to handle multiple questions and translation requests can become second nature.

Case 4.3. Two months after the original request, an Alzheimer's disease/dementing illness informational meeting was held at the Navajo Reservation Meeting Hall. It had taken that long for the agency professional to find a replacement for the original member of the agency bicultural-pair team. A member of the Indian Community Center volunteered to assist. The arrangement was that the Indian Community Center staff member would get the meeting started. Then the practitioner would begin to offer the Alzheimer's disease content allowing the bicultural team member to translate. Even though both had gone over the content before the session, it was clear that the Navajo language did not have exact terms for some of the information.

In the course of the presentation, some of the younger family members addressed their questions in English. These interchanges of course had to also be translated back into Navajo. During the informal coffee time that followed the talk, some of the family members who came up to the bicultural team spoke primarily in Navajo; others spoke English. The bicultural team found little time to socialize as the members had to call on each other for assistance in responding to the many additional questions that came their way.

Obviously, there is much more to the initiation and refinement of the bicultural-pair than can be detailed in a brief case study. Sometimes it takes time to locate a suitable bicultural member of the team. Advance preparation will serve the team well, although there is always the possibility of some rocky moments as it appears that the information is not getting through in the audience's native language. However, there is always the opportunity to recast or repeat the message from another angle. Moreover, even when sessions may be planned to be conducted in the ethnic group's language, the bicultural-pair team must also be alert to respond to the requests coming in English. Finally, even at the social break time there is no relaxing. The intercultural team is there to provide information and guidance throughout the whole event. When involved in the field setting and engaged in the task of providing information and interacting with the target ethnic group members, practitioners need to remain interculturally alert at all times.

More will be said about the concept of the bicultural-pair in Chapter 11 with reference to the cultural broker role, which the bilingual/bicultural members of the bicultural-pair team perform. At present, the central issue is that the monocultural English-speaking practitioner and the bilingual/bicultural member of the bicultural-pair team need to go through a formation period that includes comprehensive preparations for working with dementia-affected ethnically diverse clients. It should be recognized that this expectation is no different than that already indicated regarding the advance preparation needed by the fully bilingual/bicultural professional working alone. The difference is that the bicultural-pair is preparing for two. Moreover, practitioners will find that as the members of the bicultural-pair work together consistently, much of the preparation time will be cut short, and eventually an easier joint working style will develop. As an end product, a bicultural dementia-knowledgeable team will be formed. This team can eventually be seen as an overall cost-efficient approach to cross-cultural service, despite the seemingly high, up-front expenditure of sending two persons out to the same site, as well as the labor-intensive initial learning curve feature of the effort.

CULTURE-FAIR COMMUNICATION

Practitioners who are familiar with communicating across languages know that it is all too easy to fall into direct translations of the more technical aspects of the content, such as occurred in Case 4.2 with the Padilla family. There, the Alzheimer's disease/ dementing illness message, although medically correct, became too complex for the family members. They did not normally use the term *cognitive impairment*. Professionals and providers, whether working as bilingual practitioners or as members of a bicultural-pair, must therefore be certain that the context and meaning of the intended message is communicated in an equivalent understandable level in the client ethnic group's language. The initial exchange by the nurse in Case 4.2 was an accurate enough translation, but not a culture-fair communication to the Padilla family. Once the nurse considered the impact of her first effort she switched to a *culture-fair* communication approach (Valle, 1990a, 1994). In culture-fair communication communicators, instead of *translating* the information, *transculturate* it, that is, they search for an equivalent way to get the original core idea (or construct) across in the appropriate language. As indicated, more will be said about transculturating messages and communications in Chapter 12. For the moment what is important is to make certain that one is communicating in a culture-fair manner, that is, the communication, especially around dementing illness, must remain "technically sound" but made understandable in the linguistic style and at the level of comprehension of the target audience.

The idea of assuring culture-fair communication places the responsibility on the part of the bilingual/bicultural practitioner and/or the bicultural-pair to be familiar with the local language norms. As noted in Chapter 12, acculturation pressures and the presence of new arrivals to the ethnic group tend to cause shifts in the traditional language. Such variations often show up in regional differences so that even the most bilingual professional or provider has to engage in a refamiliarization with the local idiom when entering a new setting where the ethnic group's common language may prevail. The notion of assuring culture-fair communications also alerts the practitioner to possible pitfalls in exchanging information where the two parties may be far apart with respect to the technical aspects of the intended message. Finally, in mixed audiences where both English and the native language prevail, as well as in situations where the audience is composed of both lay and technically prepared persons, the idea of culture-fair communications helps the practitioner to be able to respond at several different levels in the same session. In Case 4.3 the members of the bicultural-pair found themselves communicating with both English- and Navajo-only speakers in the audience. The nurse in the case of the Padilla family (Case 4.2) found herself between the physician's medical diagnosis and the family members' level of understanding.

Culture-Fair Exchanges and Communication Theory

It might also be useful to expand the discussion of culture-fair communication and integrate it with some of the basics of communication theory. Irrespective of ethnicity, messages and communications can be broken down into a series of steps or phases, as indicated in Figure 4.1 (Braun et al., 1995; DuBrin, 1974; Samovar & Porter, 1995). As indicated by the preceding authors, each element of the communication process plays an important role in how the different parties understand each other. Summarized here, these phases include: (a) the stimulus for the communication; (b) the encoding of the message; (c) its actual transmission; (d) through some medium; (e) its

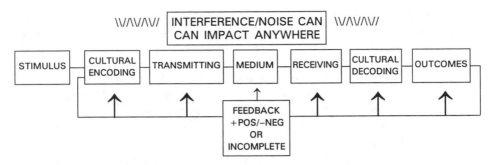

The communication process is cyclical, with positive, negative, or incomplete feedback affecting all aspects of the process.

Stimulus	The event or circumstance that causes the message to be initiated.
Cultural encoding	Begins when the *sender* perceives an experience, or multiple experiences, and *formulates* a series of symbols for expressing these experiences/ messages. These messages can be cast into *high-* and *low-*context communication formats.
Transmitting	The encoded message is then *directed* to the intended target, which can be individuals, groups, or present or absent audiences.
Medium	The message is processed through a *channel,* which can include visual, verbal, and/or written formats as well as a variety of media, including print, audio, video, and the emergent electronic *channels.* It can include such settings as a family conference or a presentation before a larger audience. The medium permits various formats to be used simultaneously, for example, the presentation could be televised, a radio talk could have callers, and so on.
Receiving	The message is *gathered* by the target audience, which has its own unique receptors at different levels of functional readiness and capability.
Cultural decoding	The message is then passed through the target audience's ethnocentric/ culturecentric decoding filters. The recipient's physical functioning capabiltiies and psychological states also come into play. Successful intercultural communication occurs when the *decoding* of the *message* by the *receiver* matches the *encoding* by the sender.
Feedback	*Back-communication* to the *sender* can occur anywhere along the communication chain. For that matter, back-communication can come to anyone along the communication chain or to any part of the chain. The feedback can be solicited or unsolicited. It can be positive, or negative. The feedback can be *intelligible,* or it can take the form of *noise, static,* or *interference.*
Interference and noise	Interference with the message can occur anywhere along the line in the communication process including the feedback that comes back through the lines of intercultural communication effort.

Sources: Modification of models by DuBrin (1974) and Samovar and Porter (1994).

Figure 4.1 Intercultural communication process model.

reception; (f) its decoding by the recipient; (g) the feedback process; and (h) the recognition that "noise" or interference can occur anywhere along the process, especially when the communication exchange is crossing cultures with different values, beliefs, and attitudinal orientations operating.

In the context of the actual communication process, the different steps take place very quickly between the initiator of the message and the person(s) receiving it. In fact, communication events happen so swiftly that the people communicating are scarcely aware of all the steps involved. Looking at the model from an intercultural engagement/culture-fair communication viewpoint adds to the importance that professionals and providers need to give to the messages they construct and exchange with ethnically diverse clients (Taylor, 1992).

In the first case discussed in this chapter (Case 4.1, the López family), the *stimulus* for the communication exchange was the fact that a diagnosis had been made. The *encoded* message was the diagnosis of Mr. López's dementing condition as having a venereal disease origin. The *transmission* was made by the monocultural English-speaking clinic staff member communicating the diagnosis. The *medium* was the exit conference setting. The message *recipient* was the bilingual daughter. However, from that point on the original message was dramatically changed because of the emotionally charged nature of the information. Mr. López's dementia was of a sexual transmission origin. At the point that the daughter *decoded* the message she did not think it culturally correct for her to communicate what she considered content inappropriate to her role. Instead she recoded it for communication to the family in what was to her a much more role-compatible and culturally accepted form. The problem was that the recommunicated message, although put into the family's communication idiom, was incorrect. *Noise* and *interference* had entered into the intercultural communication process through the manner in which the family go-between–*communicator–translator* interpreted her role and what she thought was appropriate for her to relay to her mother.

The *feedback process* actually took some time and had to wait for the clarifications of the bilingual/bicultural staff member who had been on leave. Applying the intercultural communication model in Figure 4.1 to the López case in a retrospective manner, it becomes clear that the lack of a bilingual practitioner–communicator had a powerful effect on the intended message not getting through to the family. As a consequence misinformation circulated throughout the group until it was eventually corrected by the family physician's call to Mrs. López. Noise or interference can enter anywhere along the line of the communication process, particularly where different languages are involved. Interference likewise enters where different understandings of the content are present and is almost present where strong emotional reactions surface. Generally speaking, exchanges around dementing illness are generally highly charged. Intercultural exchanges about the same issues are equally powerfully emotive.

As a further set of considerations, the bicultural practitioner's exchanges with the López family members included other important intercultural communication exchanges. When the bilingual staff member returned, she had to make sure that the daughter did not lose face in the eventual clarifications that were made. Moreover, the practitioner had to make sure to communicate the sexual origins of Mr. López's dementing condition in a discreet manner, particularly if Mrs. López herself had to be tested for the presence of venereal disease. The culturally sensitive intercultural communicator can find ways to communicate the message correctly by paying attention to the subtle rules of exchanging messages within ethnically diverse populations. In the López case, had the practitioner been present, she could have taken Mrs. López aside and worked independently with her.

High- and Low-Context Communication

There is another aspect of communication theory that applies directly to intercultural exchanges and the notion of culture-fair messages. This is the notion of *high-* and *low-context communications* (Brislin, 1993; Gudykunst, 1994; Samovar & Porter, 1995). In low-context communication the intent is to include the complete message in what is written or portrayed. Here the professional or provider needs to think of technical information. The diagnosis has to be explicit. The eligibility criteria have to be precise. The intake format has to be direct and to the point. In contrast, high-context communication contains much that is implicit; that is not directly stated, and that might be expressed in symbolic form. Here one might think of a poem that is primarily evocative in nature, a painting that stimulates the imagination, or a story or fable that contains an implicit rather than an explicit message.

The intercultural connection is that many traditionally oriented cultures use high-context formats for many of their communications. They will get to their point indirectly rather than directly. The communicational exchanges are surrounded by normative expectations about the statuses or roles of the parties communicating. They also may express their ideas in more symbolic ways. To some extent the daughter in the López case (Case 4.1) used a high-context approach to communicate the message of her father's condition. She had received a low-context message—that Mr. López had a dementing condition of a venereal disease origin. Because she could not bring herself to relay the message directly, both because of her feelings and because of her cultural upbringing as the daughter in a more traditional Hispanic family, she communicated in a more indirect, high-context manner. This approach omitted vital information and was not helpful to the situation, in which the physicians were bound to report the need for Mrs. López to be tested. In many exchanges between professionals and providers, be they bilingual/bicultural themselves or part of a bicultural-pair and an ethnic client group member, there is usually much at stake. For example, the session could be determining the ethnic client's eligibility for services or, as in the López case, the meaning of a diagnostic or test procedure. The pressure for the practitioner in such communications is to keep ambiguities to a minimum. However, the ethnically diverse client coming from a high-context culture may be left waiting to see if there is more information to be imparted, or may be expecting certain courtesies to be exchanged. In the interest of maintaining a culture-fair approach, therefore, professionals and providers need to watch for signs that their clients are expecting more, even though from the practitioner's standpoint the message was clear. There may not be any more content. In such instances, one may have to repeat the same message using different terms, or approach it from a different conversational angle.

In situations in which practitioners encounter high-context cultures, they can expect that formally written messages, letters, or reports will also need some face-to-face interpersonal contact. High-context communication-oriented cultures prize the aspect of message exchanges in which the members of the group can meet to interact. In such situations, the professional or provider can follow up the formal message with a home or clinic visit, or at times a telephone call, even if this is not quite face-to-face contact. It is not that letters or reports, particularly those regarding the dementia patient's condition, should be avoided. Rather, the issue is not to expect that they will convey the total message when one is dealing with ethnically diverse populations with different communicational expectations, which often involve relational components.

> Case 4.4. The clinic had completed its evaluation of Mrs. Rowan as having probable Alzheimer's disease. Mr. and Mrs. Rowan were an African American couple from a rural area in the eastern part of the state. Because the Rowans lived at a distance, and Mr. Rowan himself was frail, the supervisor decided against asking him to return for the exit interview. Instead the clinic sent a very sensitively worded letter with information about how to get home help services in the Rowans' area. Sometime later a rural outreach worker, assigned as a circuit-rider covering the catchment where the Rowans lived, communicated to the clinic how disappointed Mr. Rowan had been with the final contact. He appreciated the written information about his wife but said he felt that the clinic was a cold place and didn't really care for him and his wife. This statement took the supervisor aback. If anything she felt that the clinic had demonstrated special consideration for Mr. Rowan. But on reflection she realized that, culturally, Mr. Rowan wanted a final face-to-face meeting, regardless of his frailty.

In the instance that the overall notion about high- and low-context communications might not be clear, the major portion of this text might be used as an example of a low-context content. It cannot depend on any accompanying body language or other nonverbal means to convey the meaning of what is being stated. The case examples used at various points in the narrative might be closer to high-context information. In the Rowan case a complex situation is being portrayed in a shortened format to illustrate the point or principle being made. Experienced practitioners will be well aware from their own circumstances that most cases are rarely simple.

Ingroup–Outgroup Communicational Considerations

Finally, to round out the intercultural communicational picture, professionals and providers need to keep in mind that, even if they come from the same ethnic group as the clients, they still remain as outgroup members until the appropriate rituals of establishing cultural rapport (discussed in Chapter 5) are observed and they are then brought closer into the target ethnic group's inner normative sphere, where their ingroup processes and value orientations operate. For example, in some ethnic groups communications with intimates and with relative strangers have different linguistic formats. Each has distinct rules of formality about how to send and receive messages. In many cultures this carries over to how individuals of different generations or social statuses within the ethnic group are to communicate with each other, so that elders are addressed differently and more respectfully than are the young.

As Gudykunst (1994) indicates, the practitioner must keep in mind that the rules that encompass the formal exchanges with strangers are less visible to people who are the outsiders—the outgroup participants—relative to the immediate culture being contacted. This circumstance often makes it more difficult to get the correct message across. In Case 4.2 (the Padilla family), even though the nurse was from the same culture as the clients, she had to reach into the speech and communication patterns of the family group before the doctor's information about Mr. Padilla's Alzheimer's disease diagnosis could get through. The professional or provider must maintain a constant awareness of the fine-line nuances in interpersonal communications in general and especially when they are crossing cultures with these communications—even if the crossing is made within their own culture.

WORKING PRINCIPLES FOR LANGUAGE ENGAGEMENT: A SUMMARY

Language and intercultural communication processes cover much ground. However there are a number of steps that professionals and providers can follow to ensure that two-way communication between themselves and their culturally diverse family clients takes place.

1. **The practitioner needs to work speedily to identify the preferred language for communication.** It may be that the primary caregiver is using the family's own bilingual, English-speaking broker for the initial contact. But in reality the caregiver and the family members may prefer that the family's native language be used from then on. The fact that the dementia-affected elder may be monolingual only with respect to the ethnic group's language also has great bearing on the situation. In any event, just as in Case 4.3, the bicultural-pair came prepared to present the content in the Navajo language but remained flexible to also use English when needed.

2. **The practitioner must be ready to expect a number of significant others involved within many ethnically diverse family situations.** Therefore, the professional or provider needs to also move quickly to relate to all those assembled.

> Case 4.5. The Alzheimer's caregiver project staff member had been working with Mrs. Gonzalez, the primary caregiver, and her sister for some time. He saw that the time had come for a family-wide conference because conflicting views of how to care for the dementia-affected family matriarch had surfaced into ongoing arguments. When he arrived, he found not only family members present who lived nearby, but also some of the out-of-state relatives, with a smattering of children and grandchildren, along with a neighbor. Recognizing this as a very normal situation to be encountered with Latino families, he moved easily into the conference with all in attendance.

3. **Although attention is paid to the need to communicate in the ethnic client group's native language, the practitioner has to avoid falling into stereotypes.** For example, assumptions should not be made that just because

the dementia-affected elder is from a specific ethnic group the professional or the provider should immediately jump into the ethnic group's native idiom. There are many aspects of linguistic analysis that need to be considered, such as the patient's premorbid original language dominance (Arámbula, 1992, p. 393).

> Case 4.6. Mrs. Garcia, an 80-year-old Latina elder of Nicaraguan heritage with a suspected Alzheimer's condition, had been tested with the Alzheimer Center's neuropsychological battery in English as a part of the diagnostic process. Her Euro-Anglo husband, the primary caregiver, and the family significant others took exception to this part of the differential diagnostic process and asked that Mrs. Garcia be retested in Spanish. A bilingual/bicultural consultant was called in to readminister the test. Immediately it became evident that, despite the fact that the patient had lived the first few years of her life in Nicaragua, she was clearly an English-dominant person and that the use of Spanish was actually fatiguing her. Moreover, when the bilingual test consultant spoke to Mrs. Garcia in Spanish, she tended to respond in English. These results were explained to the family members who reluctantly began to face the reality of Mrs. Garcia's dementing condition.

4. **One needs to always keep in mind that language is not just a verbal exchange or an explicitly written form of expression.** In the language portion of the overall cultural mapping process there is a need to observe and document the ethnic group's forms of nonverbal communication that constitute a part of their high-context cultural orientation. The elements to observe can include the following items.

   - The meaning and importance of the "affect" or feelings that accompany the communications must be properly identified. For example, the ethnically diverse client who smiles and continually says "yes" may not be agreeing or even understanding the message being given but might rather be behaving in a culturally dictated polite manner in order not to offend the other person.
   - The "body language" used within the ethnic group has to be appropriately understood. It is true that professionals and providers may be trained to recognize body language in general communication situations they encounter. However, this awareness must be broadened to become cross-cultural in scope. The refusal of the ethnically diverse client to make eye contact may not mean either resistance, fear, or subservience—rather it can be a mark of intergenerational deference, or respect shown to a person of assumed higher status, such as a professional or provider.
   - The setting in which the communication is made has to be taken into consideration. For example, an ethnically diverse client may feel ill at ease in the office interview and more at ease in their home. In some instances, given specific circumstances, these preferences could be reversed.

- The key references to stories and sayings that are used have to be incorporated into the overall picture of the patient's behaviors and the family processes. For example, some ethnic group families have "stories" or events in their family histories that have great moral influence on the present situations the members face. Observing certain celebrations and rituals can have equal communicational importance. Having these events disturbed can create considerable problems for all the members involved.

> Case 4.7. The Guerrero family members were becoming quite concerned about taking their mother, an Alzheimer's patient, to any more of their regular holiday outings or to restaurants or festivals, which Mrs. Guerrero had always enjoyed. What had begun to happen with great regularity during these outings was that Mrs. Guerrero would cry in a loud voice *"!No soy puta, no soy puta!"* ("I am not a prostitute! I am not a prostitute!"), becoming quite agitated in the process. Mrs. Guerrero's behavior seemed to intensify when she was getting dressed up and her once-favorite perfumes were used, but no one could determine what triggered the outbursts. The problem appeared insoluble. Light was thrown on the situation when Mrs. Guerrero's older sister told the story of when, as teenagers, they put on their mother's makeup and perfume and had gone to a *tardeada* (an afternoon dance in the town) without asking their father's permission. He had marched down and confronted them publicly outside the dance hall saying *"Solamente las putas se comportan asi"* ("Only prostitutes behave like this"). The family decided to try outings without the perfumes-and-dressing-up approach. They also determined to reassure Mrs. Guerrero verbally that she was not a bad person. The new approach cut down on the agitation, although perfumes from passersby still triggered some occasional reactions by Mrs. Guerrero.

5. **The professional or provider needs to observe and record the symbols that are pertinent to the ethnically diverse group's communication formats.** This includes such things as the artifacts and decorations that can be noted around the dementia patient's home, the artwork or art formats that are relevant to the group, the ethnic group's heros, and the holidays or special festivals that are observed. Walking into a more traditional ethnic Mexican American home, and later an ethnic Japanese American home, creates a quite different visual picture relative to the artifacts that adorn the rooms. The Chinese New Year and the Vietnamese observance of *Tet* have different significance for the specific ethnic group members celebrating the events, just as Chanukah, Christmas, and Kwanzaa (a winter cultural celebration becoming more widely observed by African Americans; Kwanzaa Information Center, 1997) do for other ethnics. The importance, or lack of importance, given to such events by must be logged into the practitioner's thinking. In brief, intercultural or cross-ethnic communication transcends simply knowing the group's spoken or written language.

6. **When the professional or provider is not proficient in the target ethnic group's native language, there is a need to form bicultural-pairs.** The

practitioner and/or the parent organization needs to pair the dementia-capable practitioner with a culturally competent communicator from the target ethnic group. This individual needs to be someone other than a family member. The overall intent is to serve ethnically diverse families rather than to add to the burden of individual family members.

END NOTE

Language is a vital means by which to understand another culture. At the same time, many professionals and providers find it difficult to master languages other than their own. This might appear to be a major barrier to proceeding any farther into the cultural mapping process. Not so! Language, that is, the specific sounds and symbols of an ethnic group's means of communication, is not the sole means by which cultures express themselves. As the subsequent chapters will illustrate, there are other patterns by which ethnocultural groups express themselves. Moreover, if the professional or provider has been thorough in studying the cultural–historical presence of a target ethnic group, as detailed in Chapter 3, much can be known about the group's values, outlooks, and expectations. Finally, the practitioner has another avenue through which to access the target ethnic group's language: through the bicultural-pair arrangement, discussed above and subsequently throughout the text.

Chapter 5

Interaction Patterns, Roles, and Relationships

The next rung in the cultural engagement ladder is the cultural mapping of the *pre-ferred interactional patterns* of the target ethnic group (Graham, 1993; Valle & Martinez, 1985). When engaging the more traditional, culture-of-origin–oriented client group members the practitioner proceeds to (a) clearly identify the ethnic group member's expectations about the establishment of rapport and trust; (b) be mindful that, if a bicultural-pair is making the contact, the rules for establishing cultural rapport remain the same; (c) be prepared for the presence of informal second opinions within the caregiving situation; (d) understand and be able to work within the realities of such a decision-influencing network; (e) tune into the ethnic family's help-seeking and help-accepting patterns; and (f) develop an overall repertoire of techniques for identifying the ethnic group's interactive patterns, to include the presence of non-kin (fictive kin) members (Boston, 1992; Cowgill, 1986; Elliot et al., 1996; Gaines, 1988–1989; Gonzalez, Gitlin, & Lyons, 1995; Moore Hines et al., 1992).

There are a number of specific approaches that can be used by the professional or provider seeking to understand the relational patterns of the target ethnic group. In moving the intercultural engagement process ahead, the professional or provider remains alert to how the family relationships and friendships are played out within the ethnic group itself. The practitioner also examines how the ethnic group members formulate their relationships with *strangers* or outgroup members (Cushner & Brislin, 1996; Gudykunst, 1994).

From a cultural standpoint, professionals and providers must recognize that, at the onset, they are outsiders and strangers to the target ethnic group. Being from the same ethnic group gives the practitioner somewhat of an edge. But regardless of whether the ethnic ties exist, practitioners must be knowledgeable about the *cultural etiquette* for initiating and maintaining relationships with ethnically diverse clients and patients. The rules for practicing this cultural etiquette must be observed implicitly as they are rarely explicitly stated. Perhaps they might be explicitly communicated in background documents or in intercultural briefings about an ethnic group being targeted for services, but not in the interactive situation itself.

It is here that the approach outlined in Chapter 3 of knowing about the cultural–historical ethnic group being targeted for services comes into play. A working familiarity with the group's preferred language and communication style as detailed in Chapter 3 either as a bilingual/bicultural professional, or as a member of the bicultural-pair, is indicated.

CULTURAL EXPECTATIONS ABOUT RAPPORT AND TRUST

As a starting point for entry into the target ethnic group's network of relationships and relationship formation processes, the practitioner must understand the rapport and trust expectations of the group's members. This means that the professional or provider must be able to identify the *cultural signposts* for establishing trust even where they may be only indirectly indicated. In meeting such expectations the practitioner must therefore develop the types of observational skills that can focus on individual as well as group behaviors.

Because the assumption is that the professional or provider is basically an outsider to the ethnic group members being targeted for services, a practical first step is to be alert to the *cultural protocols* for communication between strangers. For example, when one is using a group's native language, the appropriate use of formal and informal modes of address needs to be understood, especially when one is addressing the elder members of the ethnic caregiving circle. If the practitioner is from the same ethnic group, there may be even higher expectations that the cultural protocols will be followed stringently. For example, it may be appropriate to speak in the familiar mode with children but not with the adults. Professionals or providers will be expected to be able to wait out the seemingly long and roundabout preliminary discourses that often take place before getting down to addressing the need that has brought all the parties together. What is happening at this point in the intercultural engagement process is that the ethnic group members are sounding out the practitioner to determine if this is someone with whom they can establish meaningful ties.

Practitioners should not be startled at this point in the process if they are asked seemingly personal questions, such as inquiries about their family, how long they have worked at the job, whether they like the work, and so on. Truly intimate personal questions do not enter the picture here; rather, the ethnic client group members are looking for value compatibilities wherein they can establish a deeper working relationship. Experienced bicultural practitioners and the ethnically attuned member of a bicultural-pair will recognize the boundaries clearly. For example, questions about the health of one's parents are appropriate. Questions about how the practitioner relates to them are not. Questions about what the practitioners do in their field of work are within bounds. Questions about how professionals or providers are getting on with their jobs are not. Limited and carefully timed self-disclosure is a facilitative resource in client–practitioner contacts (Ivey, 1994, p. 280).

At this phase of the intercultural engagement effort the practitioner can also comment about such items as the decorations around the house, the photographs that are noted, the weather, or make a dozen other conversational ploys. The apparent "chit-chat" has a purpose: It is a form of culturally accommodating discourse. Ethnically diverse clients have to feel culturally comfortable with the professional or provider in whom they are going to confide.

It is recognized that the process of observing the appropriate cultural protocols can add to the professional's or provider's already busy work schedule. Not the least of these pressures may come from the current parent organization itself, which often prefers much tighter practitioner–client intake or initial engagement sessions. However, the payoff in observing the culturally expected rapport-building procedures is considerable. Once in place, the cultural rapport ties do not have to be reestablished, unless the practitioner in some manner alters the original bonding. The cementing of the cultural rapport links with the initial ethnic group members has a word-of-mouth type carryover to other family members who might not have been present for the initial contacts. The observing of these processes also has considerable carryover to the development of an eventual careplan for the dementia-affected elder. However, practitioners and their supervisors cannot leave the issues to chance. There is a need to establish a service rationale for the approaches that are used. Seasoned practitioners, as well as beginning ones, must recognize that the time invested in the beginning in the establishment of rapport and trust with ethnically diverse clients can bring favorable results over time. It is wise, therefore, to record the whys and wherefores of the differences being experienced early in the intercultural engagement process, to provide documentation of the different strategies used.

> Case 5.1. The Alzheimer's agency case management supervisor was reviewing the records of the two case managers serving African American and Mandarin-speaking Chinese families in preparation for the annual service report. In both instances she noted that the intake sessions in the family home were taking almost twice as long as the those with the agency's Euro-Anglo family clientele. She was prepared for this as her own earlier work in ethnically diverse communities had reflected a similar pattern. She also felt that the upswing in the monthly census figures and the diversification of the agency's client profile would answer any questions raised at the higher administrative levels. Nonetheless, she felt it important to call the matter to the attention of all of the case managers as she wanted there to be a collective understanding among the staff about approaches being used and their justification.

There is also another level within which the cultural rapport-building protocols operate. This is in the interface between the professional or provider and the broader ethnic community as represented by its own organizational infrastructure.

Case 5.2. The governing board of the dementia-service program determined that it was crucial to undertake needs assessment of both urban and reservation Native Americans in the agency's service area for its new strategic plan. A staff member, a non-Native American with a research background, was assigned the responsibility for the task. Eager to observe the appropriate procedures, the practitioner contacted a recognized Native American cultural broker, who in turn paved the way to three tribal councils active on the different reservations as well as in the urban part of the service region where some of the Native Americans lived. Each council agreed to hear about the planned needs assessment, but none would guarantee sponsorship of the effort up front.

Over the following 2 months, the practitioner made presentations to the councils that included thorough questioning as to all aspects of the proposed project. Two more months of constant contact followed, during which decisions were not forthcoming. The dementia-service program management became concerned at the passage of time, because the strategic plan had to go to the governing board of the program. Despite the mounting pressure, the staff member felt it important not to deviate from the approach of respecting the tribal ways of arriving at decisions (Trimble et al., 1996).

At the end of this period, the eventual result was a mixed success. The urban health clinic determined that a Native American staff member would have to be trained to conduct the interviews. One of the reservation health clinics agreed that the staff member himself could conduct the dementia needs assessment interviewing, but an assigned health clinic staff person, an aide, was to accompany him throughout the interviews to make the Indian families feel comfortable. The third reservation council, with the largest health clinic, representing five tribal subgroups, declined to participate.

The short case excerpt above does not do justice to the considerable outlay of effort and patience that the practitioner used to get as far as he did. At moments it is easy for even the most experienced interculturally competent practitioners to lose heart or push too hard to obtain results. However, professionals and providers must keep themselves ethnoculturally on track. Moreover, the overall process of the meshing of normative outlooks and expectations between the practitioners and their agency on the one hand, and the ethnocultural community participants on the other hand, is one that requires time. Not only is there a there is often a steep learning curve, as was noted earlier, but there is an equally steep *interactional rapport-building curve,* which is often experienced as the members of different cultural systems—the agency and the target ethnic community—come into contact.

It is true that the organization's goal was a positive one, namely, to include the American Indian/Native American population in its service plan. At the same time the initiators of the needs assessment effort needed first to understand and work within the target ethnic group's cultural expectations. They did this by anticipating the demands of the intercultural exchange situation and agreeing to work within the ethnic group's decision processes.

However, it should be kept in mind that even careful attention to such cultural protocols does not always bring complete success. Only two of three reservation settings chose to participate. When such outcomes occur, practitioners and their superiors have to look back over the cultural–historical context of the American Indian groups, extending over 400 years, to understand the reluctance of the ethnic group members to engage in even the most worthy-appearing projects (McLemore, 1994). The practitioner must remain alert to the fact that other ethnically diverse groups may have had similar experiences. Therefore, even if the practitioner follows the cultural protocols and fails, a different impression might be left behind for other professionals or providers following a similar course of action with respect to assisting ethnically diverse populations around dementing illness concerns.

Bicultural-Pair and Trust Building

Professionals or providers who depend on the bicultural-pair arrangement will need to make certain that their culturally and linguistically attuned counterpart is knowledgeable about the subtle but real cultural expectations around relationship and trust building. It can happen that some candidates for the bicultural-pair may actually be generationally removed from their own cultures of origin. This member of the bicultural-pair must therefore brush up on his or her rapport and trust-building skills with the more traditionally oriented members of his or her own ethnic group before the team enters the field.

Skills and competencies cannot be taken for granted. For their part, monocultural English-speaking professionals or providers must acquire background knowledge about the ethnocultural group being targeted for services. In the process of forming the bicultural-pair, the monocultural practitioner should ask the bicultural-pair candidate about the key aspects of this background information. Once in the field working with the target ethnic group clients, the practitioner should ask the bicultural member of the team for briefings about the communications and exchanges that are taking place. These explanatory and clarifying briefings can take place on the spot in the field, if appropriate. They can take place back at the dementia-care organizational setting or at in-between times by phone or when traveling to and from the direct contact with the target ethnic community members.

There obviously is more to the process. Both the mainstream-culture professional or provider and the candidate for the cultural member of a bicultural-pair cannot make simplistic assumptions about the knowledge and rapport effort to be undertaken between themselves and in relation to the target ethnic community. This is particularly true with regard to dementing illness, where often so many misunderstandings about the underlying disorder may reside within the more traditionally oriented ethnocultural group members. As indicated at the onset of this discussion, these ethnic groups may be on the outside of the sources of information available to mainstream U.S. English speakers. At the same time, although every effort must be made to get the needed and correct dementia-focused information to the group members being targeted for intervention, the cultural protocols just outlined must be observed so that intercultural rapport and trust can be built.

There are other background steps the monocultural English-speaking member of the bicultural-pair can take to know if the bicultural team member meets the necessary criteria for participation in the bicultural-pair. For example, the candidate's community credentials can be checked just like any other organizational candidate's references. Before being incorporated into the bicultural team, the candidate can be invited to make a presentation on the cultural aspects and expectations of the ethnic group being targeted for services. The candidate and the practitioner can initially visit an ethnically diverse family in which one of the members is bilingual. An independent checkup can be made with the bicultural family member as to the satisfaction levels of the bicultural-pair's work in the session. Also, it is essential that the bicultural-pair candidate be seen as "neutral" relative to the members of the target ethnic group community. Actually, a better way to state the issue is that the candidate must be seen as equally invested in the welfare of all of the group members involved, especially the dementia-affected elder. It is a stereotype to indicate that all ethnically diverse families or communities are united. Factionalism exists, as do different interests. The bicultural-pair candidate must be regarded as a neutral rather than as a family or community "political ally" of one side or another. If this occurs, or if the practitioner and the parent dementia-care organization are not sensitive to the issue, then rapport and trust may be compromised.

Dementia-service organizations have a number of procedures for monitoring and assessing the practice capabilities of their staff as well as their impact on the community or their service catchment. These tools can be adapted to the bicultural-pair intercultural engagement process. Dementing illness presents many complexities and stressors for the affected families. Interventions to reduce this stress, whether they are provided to mainstream or to ethnically diverse populations, cannot be taken at their face value. Intercultural capabilities have to be assured up front.

Language of Rapport Building

Many ethnocultural groups not only have procedures for establishing trust and rapport, but they also have specific terms that best describe the quality of these kinds of ties. For example, Latinos emphasize the idea of *confianza*. For this ethnic group, this term implies much more than simple "confidence" that the relators may have with each other. The notion of *confianza* carries two additional connotations. First, it says that the two former strangers have established proper rapport, that is, there is an acknowledgement that the professional or provider has followed both the explicit as well as implicit cultural expectations for "getting down to business." This is to say that the practitioner has culturally accommodated the ethnically diverse client group, observing the already-mentioned initial conversational courtesies and communicational side discussions.

Second, the term indicates that the two former strangers are now engaged in a mutual trust relationship. Here the professional or provider must prove "true to the given word" throughout all of the subsequent phases of the relationship established between the practitioner (and/or the intercultural pair) and the dementia-affected elder's family/significant others caregiving network.

Establishment of *confianza* does not mean that all problems are solved, or that the professional or provider is always bringing only good news; rather, the meaning is closer to the understanding that the family and the professional or provider are now committed to each other in the mutual task of working together to find some relief for the dementia-affected elder and the caregiving family members. Although a Spanish-language term for rapport building and trust (*confianza*) has been used, it must be noted that the concept of rapport building also extends to other traditionally focused ethnocultural groups. Elliot et al. (1996) speak about *guanxi,* or the establishment of trusting and reciprocal relationships among the Chinese. In Tagalog Filipinos speak about reaching the highest level of interaction, or *Pakikiisa,* oneness and complete trust (McBride & Parreno, 1996), or *pakikisama,* smooth companionship (Mayers, 1980, p. 93). The Japanese may refer to *makoto,* or sincerity (Sokolovsky, 1990, p. 209). It is important that the bicultural practitioner and the bicultural-pair be alert to the language of rapport building as it applies to the specific ethnic group being targeted for dementia-care services.

PRESENCE OF "INFORMAL" SECOND OPINIONS

The process of establishing rapport with ethnically diverse families also requires close attention to the way in which the family members arrive at decisions. The professional or provider has to be alert to the fact that most often they are not just working with the primary caregiver alone (Bedolla, 1995). This leads to one of the elements of working in ethnically diverse communities that can often frustrate the practitioner. A pattern frequently evidenced by the more traditionally oriented ethnic group caregivers is that of constantly checking around with a wide range of significant others, family members, friends, and even neighbors, looking for assurance and suggestions about the decisions the practitioner may have made regarding the care of the dementia-affected elder. As can be expected in such situations, many contradicting views are forthcoming (Montalvo & Gutierrez, 1989). Moreover, considerable time may be expended by the caregiver without much evidence of progress in resolving the identified problems.

Meanwhile, the practitioner, who may be coming from a framework that looks to reducing extra client time expenditures, may be feeling additional pressure to bring the situation to closure. The complexities of putting a dementia-assistance careplan together are difficult enough, and yet the caregiver seems to be engaging in a search for informal second opinions within the extended significant-other network. Still, the practitioner cannot directly set time limits on the process.

Case 5.3. The Latino practitioner had been working with Mrs. Garcia for some time after her husband's diagnosis of Alzheimer's disease. The focus of the sessions had been around understanding Alzheimer's disease, laying the groundwork for a long- term careplan. The practitioner also had been trying to get Mrs. Garcia to take action on some of her husband's medical and dental needs before his overall condition got worse. On the practitioner's next scheduled visit to the caregiver, Mrs. Garcia turned to her and said. "I talked to a friend of mine who said her father suffered from this disease and the family took him to a curandero (an indigenous healer in the Hispanic community). The curandero did his healing and her father was cured. I am going to take my husband there."

There is no question that families of all ethnicities hold out for any glimmer of hope that the degenerative progression of Alzheimer's disease can be halted and that the patient will somehow be cured. Mrs. Garcia in Case 5.3 had these hopes. What is important is that these attitudes and expectations be addressed so that intercultural engagement progress and the rapport that has been established be able to continue.

What can happen among the more traditional, culture-of-origin–oriented family members, however, is that they will cling longer to their long-held beliefs and cultural coping patterns for reaching closure on important decisions and search farther and farther for solutions. The cross-cultural comparison here is that, just as in mainstream medical services Alzheimer's disease is diagnosed by excluding all possible alternative solutions, so do traditional cultures go through their own alternative solution exclusion process. Although the Alzheimer's condition in Case 5.3 would not be reversed by the indigenous healer, it could be that the curandero would at least help the caregiver herself by providing a culturally reassuring ritual. At the same time, the practitioner working with Mrs. Garcia recognized that valuable time was being lost in providing for other aspects of the patient's health needs. Therefore, in the interests of preventing further care delays, he bargained with Mrs. Garcia: He approved of her going through the visit to the traditional healer, but he established an alternative plan of action to begin taking care of Mr. Garcia's attendant health problems.

Practitioners will find many variations on the same theme throughout traditional cultures. They all amount to the same thing, in that many cultures have patterned ways in which "second opinions" are solicited. On the surface the processes may produce doubts and delays in getting the dementia-affected elder into a more comfortable and appropriate caregiving situation. However, they are also a way of testing the efficacy of the professional's or provider's approach against what are to the ethnic group members customary ways of doing things. With patience, the practitioners will find the ethnic group members willing to try out their suggestions.

The "bargaining" that took place in the Garcia situation is one approach to take. Another might be modeling the intended action. For example, ethnically diverse clients who have been unconnected with the mainstream of dementia services may simply be hesitating because they do not know how to make the appropriate linkages, even when told. Here the issue may not be so much a cultural belief but rather the ethnic family member's isolation from formal service systems. Whichever the source of the caregiver's hesitancy, in the early stages of careplan implementation the professional or provider may have to directly show the caregiver how to make a call to a referral agency by doing so in the caregiver's presence. This can give the ethnically diverse caregiver the opportunity to hear the kind of questions to ask and the necessary documents to assemble before going to the service organization in person. The practitioner might also have to assist in the first visit with the agency that is contacted, even if it is just meeting the family when the members get there.

It may be of concern to the practitioner that the "second opinions" that are obtained by the ethnically diverse caregiver may reflect incorrect information about dementing illness. However, it is crucial at this juncture in the establishment of intercultural relationships that the professional or provider restrain the impulse to "jump in" and set the dementia record straight. Yes, statements can be made that reflect the reality of the incurability of Alzheimer's disease. Interventions can be made to guide the care that must be provided toward more effective strategies. However, a more culturally compatible approach for the practitioner to take is to actively listen not just to what is actually being said but also how it is being said. It is also important to know who in the network is doing the talking or questioning, as well as what roles these persons play within the care situation.

To the interculturally astute practitioner, indigenous "second opinions" can provide much information about the cultural orientations of the ethnic group members. These processes allow the professional or provider to read between the cultural lines of what is being said. It may not be that the caregiver is questioning the practitioner's goodwill; rather, the caregiver may be accommodating the decision process used within the extended family group. It could also be that the caregiver is having trouble accepting the implications of a brain disease with no known cure. It could likewise be that the caregiver has accepted the inevitability of the disease process. However, other members of the family's opinion circle might still be in denial. For the moment, these significant others may be influential enough to block the caregiver from taking the necessary next steps to improve the caregiving situation. Any or all of these personal, interactional, and group belief factors may be involved at any one time. It will be up to the practitioner to decipher and distinguish which predominate within each specific intercultural situation.

Basically, professionals or providers working in the cross-cultural arena need to take into account several working assumptions. First, during the preliminary stages of the establishment of a relationship with ethnically diverse populations, they are being tested for their understanding of the target group's cultural ways. They may also be undergoing testing as to their persistence and commitment to helping meet the elder's needs. Therefore, from a cultural and interactional perspective, what is important is that professionals and providers listen with their inner cultural ear to the context of what is happening in the situation in which they are working. Second, the practitioner needs to keep in mind that the caregiver is acting out of lifelong enculturated patterns that have been ingrained within the cultural traditions of a particular ethnic group. Third, it can also happen that in some cases there is a total lack of willingness to cooperate on the part of the ethnic client group. Ethnically diverse families, just like mainstream families, sometimes make choices to take no action at all and just let the situation continue as is. However, from the intercultural engagement perspective one needs to first rule out all other cultural communication and contact difficulties before arriving at this final conclusion and subsequently stepping out of the dementia-care picture with an ethnically diverse family group that does not want to move farther at the moment.

The suggestion made throughout the cultural mapping process of gathering pertinent culture-specific information about the ethnic group's outlooks, particularly in regard to help-seeking and help-accepting behaviors, can be put to good use throughout all of the issues previously discussed. Even in the best of intercultural relational circumstances, where the practitioner's cultural acuity is operating at the maximum, it must be remembered that traditionally oriented families do not necessarily want outsiders to know what is really going on—even if they are at the edge of desperation. Given time, however, the caregiver and the family group may allow a professional or provider to help them. The establishment of rapport in a manner compatible to the ethnocultural group being targeted for services will greatly expedite the intercultural engagement process. Moreover, the ethnically diverse family members'/significant others' "feelings of crisis" at the time rapport is built and help is extended may propel the them to new perceptions of coping that would be introduced by the practitioner. There is always the possibility that the crisis could overwhelm the ethnic group members. Much will depend on the practitioner's as well as the bicultural-pair's dementia competence and cultural capabilities.

Realities of Decision-Influencing Networks

Despite the frustrations that the practitioner may experience, and as strange as it may sound, the most direct route to a culturally compatible careplan is the in-depth cultural mapping of the caregiver's decision system. This involves not just identifying the key actors but also determining whether the network members' ties as well as advice are positive or negative. Among many ethnically diverse families, the individual, to include the primary caregiver, may be ranked second in adhering to the group process itself.

The ability to recognize that many of the world's cultures place a higher value on the group, or on the family–clan–extended-kin network, is a step forward in the direction of intercultural communication and engagement (Gaines, 1988–1989; Sokolovsky, 1990). Recognition of this dynamic may be more difficult for practitioners coming from U.S. mainstream service organization culture where they are trained to identify individuals and individual need, although if professionals and providers reflect on many aspects of host society processes, the ascendancy of the group or community orientation over individual concerns, or referring back to the family group instead of just to the individual member, may not be so foreign to parts of mainstream U.S. culture (Keith et al., 1994). For example, within older "small town" cultures, the extended family and even the extended community often feature in the so-called individual's decisions. As Keith et al. (1994) go on to say, many older people are "still embedded in diverse networks of kin, neighbors, church, and services" (p. 61). Perhaps recognition of these aspects of "American" culture can be used by the task-focused practitioner to help bridge what is often a perplexing circumstance of having so many people involved in the decisions being made. What may be even worse is that these significant other people often seem to override the efforts of the primary caregiver.

Case 5.4. Mr. Noyes, an Anglo American, had developed a strong lifelong "mountain man" style. His freelance work as a self-taught metal worker combined with a love for open spaces and living with nature had drawn Mr. Noyes and his wife to live in a small high desert town. Even after years of living in the town, Mr. Noyes was still considered somewhat eccentric and an outsider. He had become somewhat accepted in Mrs. Noyes's church because she was well liked. Subsequently, Mrs. Noyes began to drop out of customary activities and at times was seen wandering aimlessly through the town. Some of the townspeople, still thinking badly about Mr. Noyes, went so far as to voice their suspicions that he was drugging her. Although a diagnosis of beginning Alzheimer's disease had been made, Mr. Noyes's understanding of Alzheimer's was quite incomplete, and he was unable to convince the townspeople about his wife's condition. Instead they called in the sheriff. The deputy knew something about dementing illness and called an Alzheimer's clinic that serviced the area. The assigned clinic staff member subsequently set up a meeting with Mr. Noyes and the townspeople. At the meeting the practitioner made information available about the nature of the dementing illness that was affecting Mrs. Noyes. It was only after these efforts that Mr. Noyes's story was believed and some support was forthcoming from the townspeople.

As the Noyes case indicates, a good rule of thumb for the intercultural practitioner to use when working with ethnically diverse populations and/or community-based cultures is to reverse one's usual posture toward working with the primary caregiver only. Professionals and providers need to actively visualize that they are not just interacting with a particular caregiver as an individual; rather, they are most likely working with an extended group. In the above example the caregiver, Mr. Noyes, was caught in the middle of a difficult situation. He was caring for his wife the best he knew how, including doing his best to continue his occupation, which at times meant he had to leave Mrs. Noyes alone. She in turn would begin to wander. He went to some of the townspeople for help. However, they knew next to nothing about dementing illness and, still skeptical about Mr. Noyes eccentric character, developed their own interpretations. It was the Alzheimer's clinic staff member's awareness of the importance of small town's social networks that opened new doors to understanding of Mrs. Noyes's illness. Working only with Mr. Noyes, the primary caregiver, would not have been the answer.

Basically, in the approach being suggested, the professional or provider can combine the cultural mapping strategies for identifying key cultural interaction patterns and roles with what can be called an eco mapping technique (Germaine, 1991, pp. 78–82). The eco map helps one to visualize the various social network players and their relationships to each other as well as to the patient and the primary caregiver. The positive and negative associations present can also be identified. Figure 5.1 can help to briefly illustrate the technique in the context of Case 5.4.

Awareness of the quantity, the kind, as well as the intensity of the interactions among the key social network members helps the professional or provider to deal with the flood of exchanges that take place. In this manner what at first may seem to be obstacles can be turned into workable arrangements. A big part, therefore, of establishing intercultural contact is the fact that traditionally oriented caregivers may tend to avoid acting alone, that is, there is a strong pull on tradition-focused ethnically diverse people to consider the group in their decision making. It can happen that circumstances, including ingroup animosities, will force other, more individualized actions, but the residuals of group orientations may persist, even if expressed in feelings of guilt about proceeding in such a manner. The issue relates to what Gaines (1988–1989) highlights as more group or collectivist familial-ties outlooks of people who might be put closer to what this text identifies as the more traditional, culture-of-origin person (see Chapter 2 with reference to the acculturation continuum). Professionals and providers implementing the intercultural engagement approach are, therefore, faced with a challenge to clearly map out the interactive situation and to pinpoint

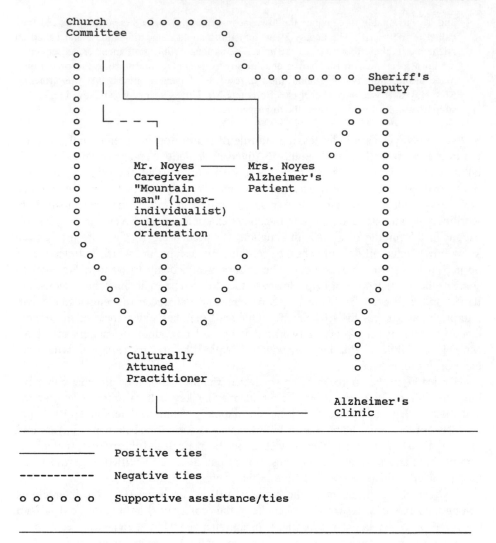

Figure 5.1 Brief ECO map of the Case 5.4 situation.

which, if any, family/significant other network members feature in the decision making about the care of the dementia-diagnosed elder. The residual concerns and apprehensions of the ethnically diverse caregiver, who may come from a collectivist background, need to be identified. This should be done as early in the situation as possible.

The presence of the decision-influencing networks in many different types of cultural situations does not mean that the practitioner must lose professional objectivity. For example, accepting the presence of a large decision-influencing circle does not mean automatic acceptance of their viewpoints. Moreover, just because the network is extensive does not mean that all of these family members, or even the network of friends and neighbors, are appropriately helping the patient or the caregiver. As noted above, with regard to the issues surrounding "informal second opinions," considerable confusion and contradictory advice may be present in the ethnically diverse client situation. Certainly for the sake of the dementia-affected elder it is important that order be introduced to the care situation.

However, in the long run it matters greatly if the professional or provider encountering different kinds of diffuse decision networks within ethnically diverse families ignores the network influentials and then proceeds to act unilaterally with the identified primary caregiver. The significant others present in the situation who influence decisions will not just go away; rather, the expectation is that they will continue to maintain either a direct or indirect voice in the caregiving situation. If the more collectivist approach to decision making among ethnically diverse families is not clearly understood and respected, the most carefully crafted careplan will most likely flounder. Moreover, professionals and providers alike can be certain that the primary caregiver will consult this decision-influencing network before taking action whether or not the practitioners approve.

HELP-SEEKING AND HELP-ACCEPTING PATTERNS

Help-seeking and help-accepting are very culturally influenced attitudes and behaviors and often follow culturally set pathways (Rogler & Cortes, 1993). They are also very personally interpreted (Nunes, 1995). Because the practitioner identifies a need, or because the caregiver may be encountering great difficulties with the care of the dementia-affected elder, does not mean that help will either be sought or accepted. Sometimes even concerned family members within a close-knit caregiving family might not by themselves be able to break the deadlock encountered. Culturally based pride, combined with personal pride, can lead to a situation that could be termed cultural paralysis with respect to accepting a careplan suggestions.

Case 5.5. Señorita (Miss) Castro, now 55, had developed severe rheumatoid arthritis at the age of 14. She had been cared for by her mother into early adulthood. Her mother had always encouraged Miss Castro to excel despite her physical impairment. This support enabled the daughter to rise to the position of office manager in a large health care organization. The mother, now 77, was diagnosed with Alzheimer's disease, and the other family members saw Miss Castro, as the single daughter, as the primary caregiver. As a traditional Latina she accepted the role gladly. She saw it as a part of her *deber* (her sense of cultural obligation) to her mother. She therefore took early retirement to take on a caregiving role for her mother. But there were severe problems, as Miss Castro was herself physically quite incapacitated and could not handle some of her mother's ADL needs, such as lifting her and bathing her. However, the daughter said nothing and did not ask for outside help. The mother fell, and the paramedics had to be called in. In the hospital the discharge planner, recognizing the dangers of the home situation, held up the mother's immediate discharge and tried to set up a different home support plan. The daughter found herself in great conflict. She felt that her family expected her to continue. She also felt it was her personal obligation. Recognizing a cultural impasse, the discharge planner called for a family conference.

As can be inferred, there was more to the Castro family's circumstances than meets the eye. Moreover, not all situations have fortuitous events that permit their partial resolution. In the Castro family situation, the discharge planner did find that because the daughter had overcome such numerous difficulties for so many years, the family members did not realize that, now in the caregiver role, she was overcompensating and placing both her own and her mother's health at risk. A rotating support plan was worked out in which other daughters and family members gave time and support to the caregiving tasks. Although this was difficult at first for Miss Castro to accept, she did see the wisdom of the recommended changes. From an ethnocultural perspective, help-seeking and help-accepting activities may encompass everything from gender-based task allocations through internalized cultural expectations of one's personal responsibilities with regard to caregiving. The acculturation continuum formulation can also be used to good effect in analyzing the attitudes and behaviors of the key persons involved in the situations. In the case of the Castro family, the daughter could be placed at the traditional end of the continuum, with the other family members somewhere along the bicultural or middle range of the continuum.

TECHNIQUES FOR IDENTIFYING INTERACTIVE PATTERNS

Observation of the interactive patterns of the ethnically diverse client group can often yield considerable information that will assist the professional or the provider to draw a more comprehensive cultural map of the important social network players involved in the caregiving situation. The various considerations covered in this chapter can be incorporated into a series of working principles, summarized as follows.

1. **The practitioner, whether bilingual/bicultural or working as part of a bicultural-pair, must observe the target ethnic group's cultural protocols for establishing trust and rapport.** Cultural courtesies have to be observed. Their observance may slow the actual service process down in the initial stages. However, if the group's cultural expectations for engaging in relationships with people outside of the kinship/significant other network are not observed and respected, the practitioner will find difficulties farther down the line in the careplanning process. In meeting these expectations, professionals and providers must be alert to pressures that may come from their own parent organization or its sponsors to move more quickly into the relationship. Here the practitioner needs to stand firm and respect what is often humorously referred to as "Jewish time," "Latino time," "Vietnamese time," and so on. The issue of ethnic group time refers to the sequence of events and process that are considered appropriate for establishing trust and rapport and that must be observed. In breaking through the seeming deadlocks between the dementia-care organization's timeliness and the ethnic group's outlooks on the process, the practitioner can apply other facets of the cultural mapping approach, such as listening for the caregiver's and the family/significant other's cultural signals that indicate that trust and rapport have been attained. Once in place, the professional or provider can then move ahead with the careplan.

2. **In targeting ethnically diverse populations, the professional or provider needs to identify and document the significant others who are involved beyond the primary caregiver.** The documentation needs to extend to intergenerational relationship patterns (Hines et al., 1992). Throughout all of this activity, the practitioner must be ready to engage multiple significant others entering the caregiving situation, rather than individual caregivers acting alone. In essence, when it comes to caregiving and careplanning situations, there will usually be a decision-influencing network surrounding the caregiver and the dementia-affected elder. These significant others could include friends and neighbors, not just blood kin. These significant others could live close by or at a distance but nonetheless remain influential within the family's decision process. The roles played by the different members of the caregiving network need to be clearly identified so that the practitioner or provider can work with the relational positives and negatives operating in the situation.

    On balance, however, the practitioner should not carry this expectation to the extreme of a stereotype so that every ethnically diverse dementia-care situation has to have multiple actors. As with other populations, some primary caregivers and dementia-affected elders will be found by themselves. However, from a cultural perspective they may still favor a collectivist or group decision process. Here the practitioner may need to become creative and simulate a process whereby the ethnically diverse caregiver can have access to some kind of second opinions so as to be able to arrive at decisions more comfortably. Facilitating the establishment of ties between the caregiver and community-based ethnically focused resources, community centers, service organizations, and local churches can assist the ethnically diverse caregiver to sometimes establish the sense of having a network that can be consulted.

3. **In connecting with the interactive patterns of the target ethnic group family, the professional or provider needs to be ready to use a combination of approaches to gather the necessary information.** Certainly, the caregiver's and the extended family group's orientations and practices can be documented as they occur. However, what is also helpful is to engage in prior preparation by means of gathering whatever information may be already available about the specific ethnically diverse client group to be served. The practitioner can also contact other knowledgeable professional and/or community informants. The various cultural–historical techniques discussed in Chapter 3 can be very effectively used by the practitioner in this background information activity, in both the preliminary and ongoing, more advanced stages of the intercultural working relationship that is formed. Considered reflection about one's own direct experience with other members of the target ethnic group can likewise be put to good use.

4. **Finally, the practitioner must identify and understand the underlying help-seeking and help-accepting orientations of the caregiver and family significant-other network members as vital components of connecting with the overall interactional patterns of the client group.** Here the professional or provider should apply the previously discussed acculturation continuum

framework to map out the dissimilar orientations of the family/caregiving network's members. The fact that the ethnic group members are residing in a host society somewhat apart from their culture-of-origin is bound to produce variations in what may at first appear to be a solid cultural front. Alertness to such distinctions will greatly assist practitioners in working through the differences noted and mobilizing the care network toward more unified action on behalf of the dementia-affected elder.

END NOTE

Immediate attention to the establishment of culturally appropriate trust and rapport enables the professional or practitioner to move within what may at times be seen as densely interactive family networks. The approach is one that successfully blends both current situational and prior cultural background information into an overall workable careplan. The alertness of the bicultural/bilingual practitioner or the bicultural-pair to all of the interactional nuances present in the client group's network brings with it several potentially positive outcomes.

First, careplanning cultural blunders can be minimized. This is to say that the mistake of stepping on toes, or ignoring key decision-influencing family members, will be avoided. Second, the initial pattern of "too many cooks in the kitchen," that is, too many people involved in the caregiving process, can be transformed into a "many helping hands" approach. Initial interference and conflict can be turned into a more collaborative efforts on behalf of both the patient and the primary caregiver. Third, recognition of the presence of different network members at potentially different levels of acculturation has great potential benefit in individualizing parts of the intervention (Kim et al., 1991). The key members of the caregiving network who might otherwise have been left out of the information and support of the careplan that develops can be included in the effort. Fourth, careful attention has to be paid to avoiding putting additional care burden on the social network or expecting the informal social support network to do the whole job (Sokolovsky, 1990). Finally, the proposed rapport building–interactional approach allows for the empathetic affirmation of cultural outlooks and practices that will enrich the eventual careplan for the dementia-affected elder. From an overall perspective, the suggested strategy guards against too-high expectations of the family network's ability to accomplish all of the caregiving tasks on its own as well as against overburdening the network (Gratton & Wilson, 1988).

Chapter 6

Values, Beliefs, and Cultural Norms

To expand the cultural mapping process, professionals and providers must tap into the ethnically diverse client group's value orientations, or explanatory models for health and illness, as these guide the group members' actions (Christman, 1977; Elliot et al., 1996; Hanna & Rogovsky, 1992; Kleinman, 1977, 1980, 1986a, 1986b; Pickett, 1993; Triandis, Kurowski, Tecktiel, & Chan, 1993). Some aspects of values and beliefs have been touched on in the previous chapters with reference to: (a) the presence of different levels of acculturation to be found among ethnically diverse group members, (b) the fact that the practitioner must be ready to engage both multicultural and ethnic-specific environments, (c) the role of language among many ethnic groups in differentiating the status of group members and strangers when addressing each other, and (d) the ethnic-distinct approaches to seeking and accepting help along with approaches to developing intercultural rapport and trust. Still, difficulties remain for the practitioner entering the values arena, difficulties that must be confronted if a comprehensive cultural assessment is to be carried out.

The problem for the professional or provider is that values and beliefs remain, for most ethnic group members, a more guarded area other aspects of their cultural orientations (Cheng, 1987). The group's language, its art, and even the members' interactional preferences can generally be directly observed. Values and beliefs, however, are privately kept. Moreover, they tend to operate at the less consciously directed levels of the individual's personality and the ethnic group's ongoing processes. None-theless, the professional or provider seeking to follow through with the full cultural mapping process must engage the target ethic group's value preferences (Cancelmo, Millan, & Vazquez, 1990; Canino, Rubio-Stipic, Canino, & Escobar, 1992; *Culture and Caregiving*, 1992).

In addressing this mandate, this section of the narrative seeks to provide: (a) an overview of the role that values and beliefs play in the everyday life of ethnically diverse populations, (b) an understanding about the important roles that the desire for privacy and the avoidance of shame play in internal family matters, (c) additional insight into the significance that maintenance of traditional roles holds for ethnically diverse groups, (d) a further orientation to the impact of normative expectations around help-seeking and help-accepting activity, and (d) a summary of techniques for identi-fying ethnic group values and normative expectations in the clinic and in the group's home community.

HIGHLIGHTING BELIEFS: MAKING A VALUES INVENTORY

Extending the cultural mapping process to the values arena, the professional or provider starts by making as thorough an inventory as possible of the target ethnic group's underlying beliefs and normative expectations, or again, explanatory models for health and illness treatment (Christman, 1977). Every attempt needs to be made to determine the target ethnic group's traditional beliefs and outlooks (Brownlee, 1978) toward de-menting illness prior to face-to-face contact. As pointed out in earlier chapters, this aspect of the proposed *values inventory* may either lack current pertinent information for the target ethnic group as a whole or contain only sketchy outlines. It is only recently that the ethnic groups outside the mainstream culture have begun to appear in the dementia-related literature, and even here the literature dealing with the value preferences of ethnically diverse populations around dementing illness has mixed per-spectives, although some patterns are beginning to emerge for specific ethnocultural groups.

For example, Segal and Wykle (1988–1989; Wykle & Segal, 1991) stress the important role of religiosity in the lives of more traditionally oriented African Ameri-can families with a dementia-affected elder in their midst. Some preliminary research among Latino populations indicates the tendency of caregivers to keep much of what occurs to themselves, and when they do turn to others, they will turn to kin first (Valle, Willis, Vega, & Cook Gait, 1994). This is particularly so with regard to IADLs (e.g., transportation, banking, paying bills, making appointments, etc.; Valle et al., 1994). Initial findings with regard to Japanese families indicates similar patterns, as does work with American Indians/Native Americans (Valle et al., 1989). However, the practitioner must note, as do the authors of the works cited above, that much of the findings reported are of a preliminary nature and should be used primarily as a guide to the values-and-beliefs arena rather than as the final statements on the issues. For the present, the professional or provider must rely on direct contact with client families with regard to identifying ethnically diverse value orientations around the dementing illness arena.

However, a different kind of difficulty arises for the practitioner in the actual face-to-face practice situation. People, whether from ethnically diverse or mainstream cultural groups, rarely conceptualize their lives in culturally analytical terms. The practitioner should therefore not expect that an ethnically diverse caregiver will say: "When working with us we presume that you will observe our customs of establishing cultural rapport"; rather, the opposite will occur. The caregiver and family members will unconsciously expect the professional or provider to know and observe the rules for establishing rapport within the family's cultural context. Furthermore, the family will notice when the stranger does not fulfill these expectations. In addition, when the expectations are not met, the caregiver can be expected to withdraw, to just suffer in silence—perhaps expressing the disappointment experienced only to other family members. These family members/significant others may in turn become equally disillusioned by the unfulfilled aspects of intercultural engagement process.

To a great extent the failure of professionals and providers to meet cultural expectations about appropriately establishing relationships around seeking and accepting help may account for a portion of the seeming noncompliance or failure to follow through with proposed careplans on the part of ethnically diverse populations. Admittedly, failed relational expectations across cultures is not the only factor accounting for such behaviors, but it is an important consideration.

From a cultural mapping standpoint, the professional's or provider's culturally relevant knowledge base is greatly strengthened by identifying the underlying values and beliefs of the target ethnic group. This aspect of the ethnic group's cultural life can also include the members' religious orientations and their impact on ethnic group members' day-to-day responses to stress.

Also, from the cultural mapping standpoint, it is essential that when professionals and providers enter the values-and-belief domain they adopt an open, nonjudgmental attitude. The communication of either open or covert nonacceptance of the caregiver's and family members' beliefs and practices is to be avoided. Traditionally oriented ethnocultural group members are quite astute in deciphering attitudes that are skeptical of their inner beliefs. Care must therefore be taken to avoid rushing in and substituting highly technical interpretations about dementing conditions; bypassing the target ethnic group members core religious beliefs and attitudes. The practitioner needs to explore with all concerned how the family's traditional understandings or customs can be worked into an overall intervention plan.

Case 6.1. Mr. Ortega's eyes lit up at the suggestion from his children that they would pay for a trip to obtain *agua bendita* (blessed water) from the principal shrine of the Virgin of Guadalupe (a religious figure of much significance for Mexican Catholic believers) in Mexico City. He returned with the blessed water for his wife, a diagnosed Alzheimer's disease patient. Each evening the water was administered after prayers and the lighting of candles. As time passed, Mr. Ortega indicated that his wife appeared *un poco mejor estos dias* (a little better these days). Objectively, neither the professional attending the family nor the other family members could note any improvement in halting the progression of Mrs. Ortega's Alzheimer's disease. However, the evening rituals of administering the blessed water had a notable calming and supportive effect on Mr. Ortega.

Likewise, many cultures hold onto similar beliefs and normative expectations regardless of whether some of the family members have received a mainstream U.S. education and are fluently bilingual.

Case 6.2. Mrs. Landis, a Sioux tribal member living in the city, had always practiced the use of traditional herbal remedies to cure her family's aches and pains as well as prevent heart, kidney, and circulatory problems. On returning from visits to her family in South Dakota she would always bring indigenous roots, leaves, and grasses that she had purchased after consultation with the natural healers of the region. From these she made concoctions for her own and her Alzheimer's-diagnosed husband's use. Her college-educated daughters, both highly bicultural, actually went to great difficulty and expense to help Mrs. Landis make these trips. They had checked with the attending physician that the natural medicines were in no way incompatible with the patient's overall care. The different family members reported that the administration of the ancient rituals brought a sense of peace to them. Even Mr. Landis, who had lost his ability to speak, seemed to enjoy the tribal chants in his native Lacotah language that accompanied healing rituals at the family gatherings.

With patience and the application of good listening skills, professionals and providers can begin to recognize the traditional beliefs and practices that may be retained by the ethnic cohort being targeted, as illustrated by the both the Ortega and Landis cases (Cases 6.1 and 6.2). It should also come as no surprise that ethnically diverse children who have received advanced mainstream educations may still want to continue to practice key portions of their ethnic group's beliefs and customs, even if it is for their parents' sake.

Unfortunately, because many values and beliefs are implicitly adhered to, rather than explicitly expressed, the unwatchful practitioner can often bypass their importance within the overall dementing illness situation. For example, the ethnically diverse client will expect to find the family's expectations and outlooks reflected in the careplan that eventually is developed. It is for these reasons that the professional or provider needs to follow through with the steps outlined earlier in the discussion with respect to developing a culture-specific knowledge base. By undertaking such advance preparation a better knowledge of what to look for will surface at the moment of face-to-face contact. The preparation will go a long way toward organizing what is being observed.

In an intercultural-practice context, the professional or provider might also consider applying the concept of cognitive dissonance in perhaps a somewhat novel and positive sense. The term *cognitive dissonance* is generally used to describe how individuals and/or groups maintain seemingly opposite, or even contradictory ideas, side by side without clear resolution. The usual examples are the discrepancies that may prevail between people's attitudes and the actions they take. In the use suggested here, the dissonance may be between belief systems and/or cognitive outlooks toward specific issues or ideas. For example, many professionally trained people from quite ethnically diverse backgrounds, including individuals from mainstream U.S. Euro-Anglo backgrounds, can hold onto both modern scientific explanations for various phenomena as well as their own personal traditional cultural or religious beliefs without major encumbrance in carrying out their professional or provider roles. A similar approach may be taken with regard to the proactive blending of traditional cultural beliefs of the family and the more orthodox medical understanding of dementing illnesses such as Alzheimer's disease.

Acceptance of traditional practices, therefore, does not preclude the application of clinical protocols for the evaluation of the elder's condition. The enhancement of the family members' understanding of Alzheimer's disease and related disorders through the sharing of medical and scientific information is likewise not to be avoided. Rather, the recommendation here is to take a step back and analyze the situation from a more objective but intercultural perspective. The professional or provider needs to examine how deeply rooted the traditional beliefs or understandings about dementing illness may be. Moreover, questions have be asked as to whether the culture-of-origin practices or beliefs are really getting in the way of a proposed treatment plan. For example, the practice of moving the dementia-affected elder among households so that all of the children can share in the caregiving can bring feelings of sharing and solidarity among the siblings. However, this arrangement may bring disorientation as a side effect to the elder. In such circumstances, the professional or provider would have to work intensively within the ethnically diverse family members' value structure to resolve the situation in the interest of bringing stability to the dementia-affected elder's living arrangements.

BARRIERS OF FEELINGS OF PRIVACY AND SHAME

Aside from deeply held religious or related beliefs, expectations around what is to be held private within the ethnic family and how circumstances considered shameful are to be handled can pose formidable barriers to intercultural engagement if not properly handled within the practitioner–ethnic group member interaction. Alzheimer's disease in particular, and other dementing conditions in general, may bring out behaviors in the affected person that are problematic, and even publicly shameful, for the family members/significant others. Cross-ethnic careplanning difficulties are only compounded when deeply held cultural values about the observance of public proprieties are seemingly violated by the dementia-affected person. Problems can often occur when family members do not understand the disease process. They may still be attaching rationality to the elder's actions, that is, they may think that somehow the actions are still under the dementia-affected person's conscious control. Careplanning is also made difficult in regard to family issues about what information is considered proper to share with others, including professionals and providers and also distant family members.

> Case 6.3. Mrs. Watanabe, an *issei* (first-generation immigrant), was beside herself. Her husband's distant cousins were planning to visit from Japan. Her husband was now more advanced in his Alzheimer's condition, and at times he would start to undress himself even in public places. Her doctor had explained that the disease process had undone her husband's thinking and his ability to control his impulses. Mrs. Watanabe also knew that Alzheimer's disease was known about in Japan. However, as she confided to her daughter, "It is still so embarrassing. Even though I tell him not to do things, he still does them.

How can we go through with the visit in his condition?" Her daughter tried to ease the situation and suggested that Mrs. Watanabe have a quiet tea for the cousins at the daughter's home and bring Mr. Watanabe only if he appeared less agitated that day. Everything possible would be done to inform the cousins about Mr. Watanabe's illness. Mrs. Watanabe agreed but still felt strong misgivings. "What will they think?" she asked. "The cousins always saw Mr. Watanabe as such an honorable person."

Assessing and then working with the elements in the Watanabe case presents a challenge for the professional and provider, particularly when he or she is working with ethnically diverse people whose traditional orientations pull them in different directions at the same time. Mrs. Watanabe wanted to fulfill her family responsibilities, while at the same time seeking to avoid public loss-of-face by having the family meeting take place in a more controlled setting, thereby also limiting family loss-of-face. However, her misgivings related to the possibility of Mr. Watanabe's personal loss-of-face remained unresolved. The factor of shame can be especially vexing for the caregiver, the practitioner, and other family members seeking to intervene, especially as its impact is often multilayered. Similarly, such situations are made even more complex by the behaviors the caregiver adopts in trying to mask the underlying situation.

Case 6.4. Mrs. Javier's switch to long-sleeved blouses in the summer and slacks along with a heavier use of makeup did not go unnoticed by her Filipino friends of long standing. When questioned about her out-of-character behavior, she would reply: "I'm doing this to please my husband." Mrs. Javier's excuses multiplied when she was asked about why she stopped attending regular social events at the local Samahan Senior Center, which she and Mr. Javier had attended for more than a decade and where Mr. Javier had been president for two terms. What was particularly telling was Mrs. Javier's failure to attend Sunday Mass, where she sang in the choir at the Filipino-language service.

Quite concerned, the parish priest made an unannounced home visit and found Mr. Javier being very aggressive with his wife, threatening to hit her. Mrs. Javier had just returned from the market, and Mr. Javier in his demented state was accusing her of visiting her lovers. Mrs. Javier managed to calm her husband enough to visit with the priest, to whom she poured out her story, even pulling up her sleeves and showing him the bruises on her arms. She also asked forgiveness for not attending Mass. The priest quickly absolved her, saying she was doing God's work taking care of Mr. Javier. He recognized that Mrs. Javier was clearly in a dilemma: She was being torn between her shame in telling the truth about the origin of the bruising and trying to prevent the shattering of her husband's good image in the community. The priest also felt that Mrs. Javier should get professional help so she could work through her own feelings.

When the presence of cultural shame is detected, such as in the Filipino cultural ambience (Mayers, 1980, p. 48), the practitioner has to remain alert to an accompanying state of *cultural paralysis* that may occur. Mrs. Javier's case exemplifies the extremes to which some ethnically diverse caregivers will go to protect the good name and status of their loved one in the community. Here the caregiver and/or the family members may be unable to act to resolve the situation in a public manner because of inner conflicts among their traditional beliefs, their status in the community of friends and family, and the patient's behaviors brought on by the disease. Mrs. Javier was, in essence, immobilized. In such instances someone from the community who is known and respected can at times break the deadlock. In the case of the Javier family, the parish priest filled this role. After some time a plan of action was worked out that enabled Mrs. Javier to break out of a part of her inaction and reopen some of her family and community contacts. Despite these efforts she still found it difficult to restart her social life.

Feelings of shame and the desire of the members of various cultures to keep problems private exert a compelling force over the caregiver's life. Sensitivity has to be shown in assisting the ethnic client to work through such deeply held orientations. Moreover, if the feelings of shame cannot be fully overcome, the professional or provider can offer some approaches to easing the inner conflicts that may be going on. In the circumstances such as just described the practitioner, by paying close attention to the cultural factors that run through the situation, can greatly assist the ethnically diverse client to literally "save face."

IMPORTANCE OF UPHOLDING TRADITIONAL ROLES

The maintenance of traditionally expected roles within the family and/or ethnic group context also reflects deeply held values. At times, despite the difficulties encountered by the caregiver, the drive to fulfill role expectations is so powerful that it is quite a challenge to assist the individual to break with personalized interpretations of her or his ethnic group traditions. Meanwhile, some family members, who may be more acculturated to the host society and who have not internalized the older generation's cultural mandates, might appear blind to the fact that the caregiver is wrestling silently to give voice to implicit cultural expectations.

Case 6.5. Mrs. Morales had been brought up in a traditional Latino family, believing that family members would care for each other throughout their lives. She had readily accepted her role of helping a variety of extended family members in times of need. She had cared not only for her own mother but also for her parents-in-law in their declining years. Now that her husband had been diagnosed with Alzheimer's disease, she began to feel that she was at the end of her ability to go on alone, but she told herself that she must. The problem was that she had always depended on her husband to drive and take care of business outside the home. Now these family matters also fell to her, and she had to constantly ask neighbors and friends for rides in their cars. She and her husband had been active with the Hispanic Senior Nutrition Center, and she had formed a close friendship with its outreach services coordinator, who still made periodic home visits to Mrs. Morales's home. At the latest visit she reluctantly confided to the director: "It's not fair, you know! Here I am, old and tired; I have to do everything for my husband and they [her children] don't help me with anything." At this point the outreach coordinator suggested a family conference might be helpful so Mrs. Morales could express her needs. Mrs. Morales declined. She said: "I have taught them just like my mother taught me. I helped her when she needed it, but my mother never had to say anything to me, I just did it. It was my *deber* (the duty owed my mother). My children should do the same."

The outreach services coordinator immediately recognized that the conflicts in the situation were very typical of many people of Mrs. Morales's generation. Mrs. Morales had internalized a lifelong role and now wanted her children to respond in the same way she did. She was hurt and even embarrassed to have brought the matter up with her friend the coordinator. Her cultural pride also had brought her to the point of cultural paralysis. The deadlock was broken as Mr. Morales's dementia worsened. The outreach services coordinator asked Mrs. Morales for permission to talk to the children. At no point in time was mention made of the lack of awareness by the children about their *deberes* (their responsibilities) or how hurt Mrs. Morales really was; rather, the focus was on formulating practical steps to better the situation.

In examining the practitioner's actions, one notes that she had made the assessment that Mrs. Morales's children, having been born and educated in the United States, had acculturated. They held different interpretation of helping roles and values than those of their mother. Moreover, they were probably busy with their lives and thought that things were being taken care of. The children were neither uncaring nor unwilling to help; rather, they had just failed to pick up on the *value nuances* implicit in the situation. Once pointed in the right direction, they collectively pitched in to help their mother. Some time later, in an exit conversation with the outreach services coordinator, Mrs. Morales sighed and said: "I know now that my children love me."

DEALING WITH NORMATIVE EXPECTATIONS

Over and above expectations about expected role performances by family members, as noted in the Morales case, cultural values and beliefs permeate the whole area of help-seeking and help-accepting behaviors.

Case 6.6. The Yee family had immigrated to the United State from Hong Kong after originally immigrating there from mainland China. The adult children were assisting their father and were quite concerned about the care of their mother, who had been diagnosed with multi-infarct dementia and was recuperating in the hospital with complications from recent additional strokes. The hospital staff, through the discharge planner, indicated that it was best that Mrs. Yee go to a continuing-care facility for some weeks of rehabilitative care rather than going directly home. The family members did not understand why she could not just come home. Two concerns emerged from the situation. First, the Yee family members were not familiar with the nature of the decisions being asked of them. Second, and even more crucial to the decision process, was the fact that the hospital staff kept bypassing their father in the discussions. The hospital had no one who could speak Mandarin, the father's native language. What was happening is that the staff kept working with the youngest adult daughter, the most fluent bilingual in the group, who was in the process of completing her university studies in the United States. However, the father felt slighted. He was the head of the family. The youngest daughter felt she was put in an awkward situation, and in the emotionally charged atmosphere could not fully translate all of the key points the discharge planner was making. The hospital staff recognized that something was amiss but could not pinpoint the difficulty.

None of the Yee family members explicitly stated their expectations regarding Mrs. Yee's care. Nor, for that matter did the acute-care facility staff; rather, both parties looked to having these unspoken expectations recognized and understood by the other. The Yees' outlook was that the family elder, Mr. Yee, would be directly consulted in the decision process. The hospital staff as a group, and the discharge planner in particular, put too much of the communication responsibility, and the apparent decision burden, on the younger bilingual daughter. It is not that the family members were failing to consider Mrs. Yee's needs; rather, they had been placed outside their customary ways of making decisions. The discharge planner, under pressure to arrive at closure, and also taking a more individual patient-oriented perspective, was not uncaring. Instead, everybody was operating on different sides of an *interactional value gulf.*

Neither side was wrong; rather, the messages from both sides, being very culturally oriented, were not being properly transmitted or received. As noted earlier, the family's orientation could be characterized as collectivist, whereas the acute-care staff could be seen as individualistic. Such cultural differences arise on a daily basis. The issue of mobilizing the hospital's resources around the needs of ethnically diverse group clients in terms of providing in-house intercultural communication capabilities requires attention, even if this might occur on a one-time-only basis. Practitioner and organizational preparedness to handle the unvoiced nuances related to ethnically diverse group members' help-accepting orientations relative to the complex arena of dementia care goes with the intercultural territory.

However, even in the absence of bilingual/bicultural staff, or of a bicultural-pair arrangement, there were some basic steps that the monolingual English-speaking discharge planner could have taken. In addition to placing the decision concerning Mrs. Yee before the family, which was done, less pressure could have been placed on the youngest Yee daughter. Time could have been left for her to step aside to let her communicate the information to the family in its own culturally expected style. Determination as to who was the principal family decision maker could also have been made by watching the affect of the family members. At times this can be inferred by watching the manner in which the family members addressed each other, especially how all might defer to Mr. Yee. In such instances, where a deficiency of language ability exists, the professional or provider can arrange the seating positions in such a way as to provide recognition of the key member's seniority. Eye contact, as appropriate, can make up for some of the lack of language capability. For example, the practitioner could have sat or stood facing Mr. Yee directly while speaking to him in English. The daughter could be placed to one side, allowing her time to transmit the message from English to Mandarin. During this time, the practitioner would focus his or her attention on Mr. Yee, only occasionally turning to the daughter, perhaps as the message from Mr. Yee would be relayed back through the daughter in English. Moments of silence and privacy could also have been used to facilitate the process. These periods take some of the pressure off of the situation in which the key individuals involved—the practitioner and the ethnically diverse client—lack the basic tool of a common language to communicate directly. There are times also when feelings can cross cultures and difficult messages can be communicated through the only person available, the family go-between. For example, the interest of resolving the problems at hand in and perhaps starting over with the Yee family, the practitioner could have inquired as to the appropriate way to express an apology to the father for any inconvenience that may have occurred and done so through the available go between, the daughter.

IDENTIFYING VALUES IN THE FIELD: A SUMMARY

A number of working principles or techniques can be put into action to concretize the values inventory component of the cultural mapping process. Despite the less visible position of values, beliefs, and normative expectations in intercultural contacts, there are ways of going about identifying these aspects of ethnic group life.

1. **As suggested in Chapter 3 and elsewhere throughout the narrative, the professional or provider must acquire some background information about the ethnic group that is being targeted for dementia-related contact.** As indicated, this activity may take the form of reading up on the ethnic group and its experience within the U.S. mainstream cultural ambience. The approach may also include seeking some form of consultive assistance from the ethnic community's cultural brokers (see Chapter 11) as well as from experienced interculturally proficient practitioners working in the dementia arena. When engaging in this acquisition of background information about the target ethnic group the focus should be on the core value–belief orientations of the ethnic group members in a variety of areas, such as the manner in which important decisions are made and the ways in which the group members seek out and make use of resources both within the family and with reference to the formal dementia-care system of services.

    To be ready to engage different ethnic group clienteles, professional and providers, as well as their service organizations, have to plan ahead to mobilize the necessary resources to obtain the group's value- and belief-oriented background information. Without this kind of information in hand, the response by the practitioner or organization at the moment of crisis might miss the mark in terms of establishing true intercultural contact.

2. **Throughout the actual interviewing/family-contacting process the professional needs to look for and identify expressions and actions that indicate the ethnic group members' underlying value and belief outlooks.** These indications can come in seemingly mundane exchanges about the daily lives of the ethnic group members, or around their preferences as to what should be done for the dementia-affected loved one, or even in terms of some culturally indigenous practices incorporating into the over-all treatment plan. To the professional or provider such cultural practices might seem unimportant and as something that will bring no inherent positive change to the dementia-affected person's underlying condition. However, to the ethnically diverse caregiver and the family/significant others, the cultural healing practices might be viewed as very substantively important and reassuring, as in Cases 6.1 and 6.2.

    It is important for the professional or provider to make certain that the indigenous practices that are introduced into the careplan remain not only complementary to the ethnically diverse client group's normative outlooks but are also conducive to what is considered appropriate dementia care for the affected person. In this latter context, the practitioner must remain alert to activities that might be counterproductive and in fact worsen the situation. When indigenous medications are introduced into dementing illness situations, it is wise to check with a knowledgeable, dementia-capable physician so as to establish an approach to monitor any contraindications to their use. Should the product being used not be easily recognized, the practitioner can consult pharmacists in the target ethnic group's community who may be informed about the properties of the substances. Libraries and the Internet are also possible resources for listings of indigenous medications used by specific ethnic groups. In addition, there are some research groups that can be consulted that focus on the differential reactions of ethnically diverse populations to medications.

3. **The professional or provider must be prepared for the fact that values and beliefs aspects of the cultural mapping process are difficult to identify in short-term professional or provider contacts.** Certainly, the hospital staff, and their spokesperson—in the Yee case (Case 6.5)—were at a disadvantage in the short time they had to understand the culture with which they were working. As discussed in this chapter and in Chapter 5, the sharing of ingroup values and beliefs with outgroup members (in the Yee case, the practitioner and the hospital staff) is a relatively guarded procedure. It depends a great deal on how the establishment of culturally appropriate rapport has proceeded. Value insights emerge over time as mutual trust is established between the practitioner and the client. The professional can augment the insights, however, by studying up on the ethnic group as a whole with repeated ongoing contacts in the community, as noted in Chapter 3. The hospital staff, or at least the discharge planner in the Yee case, could have done some on-the-spot work to at least determine what was happening. This effort, however brief in nature, might have assisted in the interaction with the family.

4. **Cultural outlooks and beliefs need to be seen as continuing over a lifetime, with one's own culture-of-origin orientations surfacing even after long periods of accommodation to a second culture.** Middle-class status and bilingual/bicultural attainments should not be seen as impediments to the retention of parallel belief systems. In Cases 6.1 and 6.2, the dementia-affected patient was not harmed in any way. Moreover, Mrs. Ortega's (Case 6.1) mental health was improved by acting on her cultural beliefs, which were present even though she had spent many years living and working in the United States. As noted earlier, the Landis case (6.2) demonstrates how both traditional and acculturated perspectives may coexist. When working with ethnically diverse groups, the professional or provider may find that traditional orientations may be "reactivated" by the exigencies of the care situation.

5. **Throughout the process of value identification, the practitioner has to be on guard against formulating stereotypes.** The professional or provider has to be cautious about extending the actions of a single ethnically diverse individual, or those of a specific family group, to the entire ethnic group, concluding that all the members think, believe, or will act in the same way. No individual or single family unit incorporates the totality of an ethnic group's culture.

The practitioner therefore has to walk a fine line between the information that is generalized about specific ethnically diverse groups. This knowledge must be put into the context of the situation at hand. Here it is especially helpful to bring in the acculturation continuum formulation (Chapter 2) and to lay out what is being observed within that context. Before making major inferences about the values that have been identified, the professional or provider analyzes and compares the information being received in the family situation with other content of a broader nature related to the ethnic group as a whole. While this is being done the practitioner looks for specific behaviors or attitudes that indicate that the caregiver's and/or the family group's underlying values are playing a vital role in their coping approaches, particularly around help-seeking and careplanning expectations.

END NOTE: VALUES AND BELIEFS DIMENSION

In sum, it is important to recognize that values and beliefs have both cognitive and affective features. The cognitive aspects are evidenced in the ethnic group's literature, its sayings, its orally communicated moral stories, and its religious documents. The affective elements are expressed in emotive and behavioral contexts. It is these that tend to predominate. Even where the ethnic group notes its values, the practitioner is still confronted with the private manner in which the individual retains values.

Despite all of these seemingly indirect aspects to their expression, traditional beliefs among ethnically diverse as well as mainstream cultural populations remain very strong influences, often guiding the caregiving individual's actions in his or her later life. Traditional values and beliefs are just as strong as the modern scientific orientations of professionals and providers. The difficulty is that the practitioner's own orientations can act as blinders. Overreliance on one's own orientations can lead to the loss of ethnoculturally significant information that may be vital to the ethnically diverse client group's dealing with dementing illness and acceptance of the eventual careplan that emerges. Information about the ethnically diverse family's underlying value sets should not be dismissed as inconsequential; rather, careful attention to the ethnic client's orientations assists the practitioner to construct a bridge between the scientific understandings of dementia and the client's indigenous comprehension of the situation. Recognizing the traditional beliefs and practices of ethnically diverse clients in no way precludes the ability of professionals to incorporate careplanning approaches that emerge from the orthodox medical and scientific fields. The bridge between the ethnic group's views and those of the field of dementia care is the interculturally capable practitioner who establishes a cultural value connection with the members of the target ethnic group.

Chapter 7

Sorting Factors Often Confused with Culture

The final step in filling out the cultural mapping process is to sort out social status type elements that can distort the cultural profile being developed of the target ethnocultural group. This chapter focuses on four factors that the literature identifies as being very often confused with the cultural features of ethnic groups and that must be distinguished (Advisory Panel on Alzheimer's Disease, 1993; Betancourt & Regeser López, 1993; Brownlee, 1978; Murdock, Schwartz, & Hwang, 1980; Mutran, 1985; Talamantes et al., 1996; Valle, 1994). Collectively, these elements include: (a) the socioeconomic status of the ethnocultural group members being targeted for services; (b) the residual effects of both past and present discrimination experienced by the group members; (c) the relative powerlessness and underclass status of the many ethnically diverse groups, which often has considerable impact on the allocation of resources and, more specifically, on the availability of and access to dementia-specific services; and (d) the level of literacy present within the target ethnic group members. To a large extent, this portion of the narrative is an amplification of the culture-distorting issues identified in Chapter 2.

It is important to recognize that the lives and social experiences of many ethnically diverse group members have been filled with stressors and illnesses beyond dementing illness itself, that is, the group members may have inordinate numbers of low-income people within their ranks. They, or members of their families, may have been the recipients of prejudice and discriminatory behaviors in both personal and institutional contexts (Alston & Mngadi, 1992), that is, the ethnic group member may have been the individual target of these types of actions, or his or her ethnic cohort may have been adversely affected by policies and practices in discrimination coming from the broader society or groups within the society. Hate crimes can be an example of personal-level actions. Discriminatory loan or job procedures illustrate the broader context of the problems encountered. Many of the ethnic groups as a whole do not have ready access to needed services, and it could be that lower levels of literacy may be found within some ethnically diverse populations. Some or all of these factors are bound to appear somewhere in the backgrounds of people who are outside the mainstream U.S. culture, although mainstream society itself does not escape from many of the same factors. For example, as noted earlier, there are extremely high functional literacy levels in the general U.S. adult (18 and over) population (*Adult Literacy,* 1993).

At the same time, the professional or provider, when entering into a discussion of the relationship of ethnicity and the various culture-distorting factors presented here, must avoid falling into stereotypes. Not all ethnically diverse groups are poor. Not all will identify prejudice and discrimination as their number-one problem. Not all are politically powerless or illiterate. Moreover, it is not just these immediately named ethnic cohorts that experience the societal processes discussed in this chapter. The U.S. society contains other ethnic groups that at one time or another may have experienced adversity. These other groups can range from the new immigrant populations entering the society, such as Arab Americans, to residents of rural communities who may be bypassed in the allocation of vitally needed services, including locally available dementia-care programs.

Therefore, from a practice and service intervention standpoint, what is needed is an approach that: (a) acknowledges the potential presence of all or any of the four elements mentioned above and (b) clearly separates them from the actual cultural assessment that is being conducted but (c) nonetheless actively integrates any residual effects identified into the total cultural mapping profile of the ethnically diverse client groups relative to dementia-care planning.

SOCIOECONOMIC STATUS CONSIDERATIONS

There is often a strong tendency to mix socioeconomic status issues with culture. It is true that a number of ethnocultural groups in the United States have a disproportionate number of low-income people within their ranks, but poverty and culture are not one and the same. In the past there have been attempts to popularize the *culture of poverty.* These approaches have only muddied the waters for the practitioner who may be trying to isolate and understand the impact of cultural factors on ethnic identity. For example, the poor people of different ethnic groups may resemble each other with respect to their low-income status. However, the poor people of each ethnic group will be found to be linguistically distinct. They will also have different value orientations and culture-of-origin reference points. Moreover, their kinship–friendship social networks will vary considerably. It is therefore inappropriate to mix income status and cultural factors into the same assessment. A sure problem for the person engaging in the cross-cultural assessment of an ethnic group is to treat socioeconomic status as a proxy for culture. An example related to the start of the national nutrition programs, although not directly related to dementia, might serve to illustrate the point.

Case 7.1. The time was the middle 1970s, after the initiation of the nutrition programs for senior citizens. In a West coast setting after a year of considerable effort, a planned-outreach program to attract low-income diverse ethnic group elderly populations, including Hispanics, African Americans, and Filipinos, was floundering. A local evaluation was undertaken to try to determine why attendance from groups other than the mainstream English-speakers was considerably lower than expected. Some of the ethnically diverse elderly who were interviewed reported that the standard American menus "were not tasty."

A pilot approach to diversify the menus to reflect ethnically varied cuisine was initiated. Consideration of certain ethnic festivities and celebrations along with the particular dishes traditionally prepared for those occasions were included. The approach began to break through the resistances that were encountered, and the participation of ethnically diverse elderly increased over the next several years. Eventually, a number of ethnically focused nutrition programs for Latinos, Filipinos, African Americans, and Jewish Americans were initiated in different parts of the region, which resulted in regular, sustained ethically diverse participation.

The actual story in Case 7.1 is more complex than as portrayed. However, what got things going in the wrong direction was the overgeneralization that because the poor elderly from the different ethnic groups might be hungry, they would all relish the same types of meals. The policy stereotype that nutrition needs could be treated the same across ethnic groups created an initial formidable barrier. It was only when diversification was introduced in the form of ethnically attractive menus and linguistically appropriate social settings that the programs became popular among the different ethnic group elderly. It took awhile for the nutrition program planners to recognize that a better use for a staple such as wheat was to permit one group to turn it into a dumpling, another into a matzo, and still another into a tortilla.

Therefore, professionals or providers building a background profile of the ethnic group or groups being targeted for services must be on their guard to avoid formulating cultural knowledge on the basis of socioeconomic status. For example, when reading about an ethnic group or reviewing planning reports it is important to check to see if the discussion is primarily about the low-income contingent within the ethnic group. What can happen is that generalizations reflective of socioeconomic need may appear to speak about the ethnic group's cultural attributes when such is not the case. Professionals and providers must be alert to the confusions that can arise even when they are talking to key informant/cultural brokers from the community. Often these brokers are faced with such overwhelming need, felt at so many levels in the community, that they too can mix economic factors with cultural attributes. Socioeconomic status generalizations will not be helpful in identifying cultural group value orientations, attitudes, and customs. Moreover, the practitioner will have to be especially vigilant to differentiate economic status information from discussions about culturally based help-seeking and help-accepting patterns.

LONG-LASTING INFLUENCE OF PAST DISCRIMINATION

Acts of discrimination experienced in the past by members of ethnically diverse groups may also have lasting effects (Pang, 1988). Current prejudicial attitudes and discriminatory experiences can likewise have powerful inhibiting effects on ethnic group members. At times it is difficult to view the daily events in the media without finding some mention of hate crimes, discrimination, or other adverse events taking place somewhere in the country, perhaps in one's own local community, directed at specific ethnic groups or individuals from these groups. However, in any cultural mapping assessment of ethnically diverse dementia-affected families, these factors, just as socioeconomic status circumstances, must be separated from cultural considerations to obtain appropriate understanding of what may be occurring in the situation.

> Case 7.2. Final arrangements had been made by the Harris family members, who lived scattered throughout the city, to place Mrs. Harris, an 80-year-old African American diagnosed with Alzheimer's disease, in a nursing home. The family recognized the need for stronger custodial care for Mrs. Harris, whose caregiver husband had recently died. None of the family members could care for her on their own, although all were contributing financially to her placement. After careful examination, a nursing home had been selected for both its well-run Alzheimer's program and for its ease of access by all of the extended family members. However, the family had one major concern: Their mother would be the only African American resident in the nursing home. Mrs. Harris's early life in the 1920s and 1930s had been filled with many traumatic events. Her parents had been among the first integrated-housing proponents of that era. They had actually been driven out of one community where their sponsors had tried to settle them, and they were "burned out" of another. Still Mrs. Harris's parents persisted. The era of World War II opened up new opportunities for the family. Mrs. Harris had become a teacher, married a college professor, and raised five children, all now in professional or business careers. With the progressive onset of her dementing illness, Mrs. Harris's recent memory was now mostly gone. She had forgotten all about the postwar events and lived mostly in that traumatic period of her early life when prejudice and discrimination came down hard on her and her family. The nursing home staff were most reassuring that all would be well, and the first few weeks proved uneventful. Mrs. Harris got into the daily routine, which included walks by neighbors' rooms. However, one day, another patient, Mr. Frederic, of Euro-Anglo background, also suffering from dementia, yelled a racist epithet at Mrs. Harris and told her to get away from his room. From that point on Mrs. Harris began to act in a fearful manner and kept saying that people were going to hurt her. She kept asking for her mother to help. These behaviors kept being reinforced as the other patient persisted in using the same epithet whenever Mrs. Harris was around. The family members noted the change in their mother and expressed their concern to the administrator, indicating that unless changes were made that they were planning to move their mother out.

The issues in Case 7.2 became quite involved for the facility, and the full solution can be only sketched out here. As Mrs. Harris was the only African American in the facility, the nursing home staff was anxious to move quickly to resolve the situation. They took several steps. Immediate action brought the family members from both Mrs. Harris's and Mr. Frederic's families together for a meeting to explain the situation. Much to the surprise of the staff, both families proved to be quite understanding and gave hints on how to work with the situation. Because both patients were cognitively impaired a training–learning action was not even considered. However, Mr. Fredric's family indicated that "Daddy has always been this way. In fact he once got into bad trouble for shooting off his mouth about blacks." They suggested that someone act the part of his old boss and tell Mr. Frederic to "quit it." For their part, Mrs. Harris's family indicated that things had gotten better for their mother when her parents had moved away from the city where their home had been burned out. The staff picked up on this and came up with a plan to simulate a move within the facility, giving Mrs. Harris a new room with a different view and furniture arrangement, and even a new walking route, avoiding face-to-face contacts between the two patients as much as possible. The family cooperated and came in for the move to a "new home." After these interventions the behaviors of both patients improved. Mr. Frederic no longer shouted his epithets. Mrs. Harris seemed very pleased to be in a "new home" and making "new friends."

Not all such situations may be able to be resolved so positively, but the case offers some insight into the powerful and long-lasting effects of racism and prior discrimination, as well as the revival of these effects by current daily life events of patients affected by Alzheimer's disease and related dementias. However, a key consideration for the professional or provider engaged in culturally mapping the situation is that the behaviors that result from events such as those just described need to be distinguished from more cultural background factors influencing the situation. The challenge for professionals and providers is to carefully distinguish prejudice and discrimination from the cultural elements discussed in previous chapters, when society as a whole still has not resolved many of these problems. But if clarity is going to be forthcoming within the cultural side of assessment, the distinctions must be made. With attention to the application of the acculturation formulation as previously outlined in Chapter 2, the practitioner can acquire the skill to make the necessary distinctions.

RELATIVE POWERLESSNESS AND UNDERCLASS STATUS

The relative powerlessness and underclass status of many ethnically diverse groups and their members can likewise affect help-seeking and help-accepting patterns (Kessler & Neighbors, 1986; Torres Gil & Fiedler, 1986–1987). These conditions also should not be confused with culture. For example, the apparent reluctance of the members of an ethnically and linguistically diverse group to engage in long-term care services cannot always be placed at the doorstep of culture. Other factors, such as the inequitable distribution of diagnostic and dementia-care resources within the community, or the relative inaccessibility of services—particularly long-term care services—may be the actual critical factors, rather than cultural beliefs and customs, that are affecting service linkage and usage for ethnically diverse populations.

If it is true that ethnically diverse populations are culturally averse to existing services and do not culturally relate to them, then one has to explain the literature that points to a different reality. For example, there are nursing homes that are patronized by various ethnically diverse populations, such as African Americans, Chinese Americans, and Native Americans (Chee & Kane, 1983; R. C. Cooley, Ostendorf, & Bickerto, 1976; McDonald-Schoemaker, 1981; Morrison, 1982; F. Novak, 1974; Sakauye et al., 1994; Schrafft, 1980; Serby et al., 1987). One also has to explain the actual presence of these and other ethnically diverse groups in day care programs and a host of other long-term care services related to dementing illness. The problem regarding the use of nursing homes may reside elsewhere and be related to the societal status of the ethnically diverse group or individual (Holmes, Holmes, Steinback, Hausner, & Rocheleau, 1979; Holmes, Teresi, & Holmes, 1981; H. Jackson, 1983; J. S. Jackson, Burns, & Gibson, 1992; Torres Gil & Fiedler, 1986–1987). For example, the utilization problem may be a consequence of the way dementia-care services are arranged, specifically with regard to their availability, their accessibility (e.g., the proximity of the service to the target ethnic group), and/or their adaptability to the target population. It can be helpful here to examine two of the factors noted, namely, the availability and accessibility of services (Wallace, 1990; Wallace, Campbell, & Lew-Ting, 1994). If one examines the regional service directories of most areas of the country, at least on paper, one perhaps can find a number of long-term-type services that indicate that they relate to specific ethnic groups. These services may even indicate that they are linguistically and culturally appropriate to the target ethnic group. There may, however, be a catch in the arrangements relative to dementing illness. For example, there may not be a culturally appropriate dementia-specific diagnostic clinic, or a community-based day center or respite program near enough to be used. As suggested earlier, it may be that the ethnic group members themselves are outside the dementia-resources information-dissemination loop. Perhaps also, despite what is said on paper in the regional directories, the services themselves are somewhat oblivious to the ethnic populations in their midst, or perhaps the service providers themselves are in a quandary as to how to conduct outreach to include the group members in the programs.

It could also be that because of their relative *cultural invisibility,* the ethnocultural populations from the region may be overlooked. Still another different factor may be at work. Because of the lack of sufficient bicultural personnel, including the lack of sufficient bicultural-pairs discussed in earlier chapters, the target ethnic group members may find themselves being relegated to a lesser level of dementia service. For example, there may be a lack of sufficient culturally and linguistically capable technical or professional diagnostic personnel on board. In such instances professionals and providers may be depending on lower level skilled personnel to act as communicators and "surrogate evaluators." In contrast, patients and caregivers from the mainstream English-speaking culture may have access to highly trained professionals who not only speak their language but who are also generally in tune with their beliefs and customs.

Therefore, before the label of *cultural barriers* is placed on the relative inability of a target ethnic group to link to and access long-term care services, several factors need to be examined independently. The members of the group may simply not know about the dementia-oriented services. They may inaccurately assume that they are ineligible for such services. The dementia-specific services may have no outreach to the members of the target ethnic group. It is equally likely that the programs that exist have given thought to outreach but may actually consider the members of the ethnic group to be an afterthought, and be providing only a sort of "second class" service to the members. All of these factors stem from social status considerations, taken either singly or in combination, and may be influencing the nonparticipation outcomes. Cultural attitudes may be a secondary consideration given the levels of need coming out of the elder's dementing condition. The case below may help illustrate some of the problems, aside from culture, that ethnoculturally diverse groups encounter in the resource-distribution arena.

> Case 7.3. It was clear to the Japanese Service Center that there was a definite need for the establishment of an Alzheimer's disease support group. More and more members of the local Japanese American community were coming forward with problems related to dement-ing illness. The center director noted that even some of the more traditional *issei* (first-generation) members were quite overwhelmed by the problems of their dementia-affected family members. The caregivers were overcoming their usual reticence and were openly asking for help. The director of the center did not know much about the disease but scheduled a talk by a Japanese American neurologist that brought out many interested people in the community, even though at the time the director had no staff member who knew enough about dementing illness to provide an ongoing service.
>
> Recognizing the need, the director called a local Alzheimer's-focused group that expressed interest along with a willingness to help. However, at the time the Alzheimer's group did not have anyone fluent in Japanese who could serve as a group leader. The Alzheimer's group offered to train any bilingual/bicultural Japanese American professional or layperson who would come forward as a Japanese support group leader. However, they could not undertake the outreach themselves.
>
> Eventually, the Japanese Service Center director was able to employ a dementia-capable professional who took on the task of not only initiating ongoing Alzheimer's dementia support group services but also of engaging "politically" within the broader Alzheimer's disease and related disorders provider–volunteer network. In this latter role she continued to bring forward not only the interests and concerns of Japanese Americans but also the issues of other Asian American populations who are affected by dementing illness.

Despite a willingness to help the Japanese American community, as outlined in Case 7.3, a direct response in the form of starting up support group services could not be undertaken by either the volunteer organization or the Japanese Service Center itself at the point in time that the needs manifested themselves. Subsequent efforts enabled the startup of a specific program for the Japanese American community. The newly hired Japanese Service Center bicultural dementia specialist was invited into the area wide multicultural committee. Regrettably, this kind of readiness is not widespread enough yet to handle the growing need for dementia-related services for all of the culturally diverse groups currently experiencing an ongoing need for culturally relevant programs and assistance.

IMPACT OF LOW LITERACY LEVELS

Cultural assumptions also need to be checked out when low levels of literacy are encountered (Valle et al., 1994). The problems of ethnically diverse caregivers relating to dementia-focused service plans may not at all be based on cultural expectations; rather, the situation may be one in which the caregiver or the family/significant others featuring in the care of the dementia-affected elder cannot handle the literacy level of the dementia-related service information that is available. Some professionals and providers do not realize that much of the technical information they disseminate describing Alzheimer's disease and related disorders is geared to a more "formally schooled" clientele.

What often occurs is that in the rush to make the information culturally relevant, this information is then translated in a relatively verbatim manner into the target ethnic group's native language. At this juncture three things happen. First, the original content is most likely pitched at too high a technical level. Second, when the content is translated into another language there is a tendency among the translators to take the material to an even higher level of schooling in the native language rather than to go the other way, toward the day-to-day idiom of the target ethic population. Here the translator may be looking to use what would be considered a proper grammatical format instead of trying to communicate the message in colloquial language. Third, the native language of the target ethnic group itself, whether colloquial or formal, may lack the equivalents of technical terms that, after all, have been developed in English. As noted earlier in the discussion, Alzheimer's disease bears the name of its discoverer, Alois Alzheimer. Moreover, whatever language is used, it must be emphasized that Alzheimer's disease as well as several other dementing conditions are diseases that affect brain function.

Without extending the discussion inordinately here, what is important to recognize is that *functional literacy* (the ability to read and comprehend messages and/or to complete required forms) rather than the culture orientation of the ethnic client might be influencing the ethnic group members' nonresponsiveness toward engaging formal dementia-related services. It may be that functional literacy (Heisel & Larson, 1984), rather than culture, is blocking the ethnically diverse group members' understanding of their family member's dementing illness. Therefore, as explained in more detail in Chapter 12, messages and information about dementing illness communicated to ethnically diverse populations must be made *literate-fair* as well as *culture fair,* that is, the communications have to be pitched at the level at which they can be understood by the target ethnic group family members as well as put into their preferred language formats.

Case 7.4. The organizers of the Alzheimer's disease community information meeting, specialists with a number of years of experience in working with dementia in the Latino community, were reviewing the previous evening's session with the staff of the Latino Community Health Clinic, which had hosted the event. The formal part of the presentation had gone well. Many of the members of the audience had asked the kind of basic questions that indicated they had become personally interested and involved. The educational caregiving video had been a boost to the presentation. The Latino Community Health Clinic director made a special point, noting that the Spanish-language *Alzheimer's fotonovelas* (pictorial magazines, popular among Latinos, that primarily show a story rather than tell it in words) had been snatched up by the audience at a much higher ratio than the conventional pamphlets in Spanish. The meeting organizers had been well aware in advance of the session of the low levels of formal schooling in the potential audience. They had reviewed the clinic's service catchment data and had come prepared with the appropriate information and communicational tools that relied more on visual than written content.

The application of the cultural mapping technique, as noted in Case 7.4, of linking to the target community's historical–demographic presence, enabled the session planners to select the appropriate materials for the educational session (Alzheimer's Cross Cultural Research and Development, 1992). Had they gone to the Latino Professionals' Conference, or to a Latino college group association meeting, they would have taken other, more elaborate or technical materials with them. They might have brought the *fotonovelas* along, but these would have been used to show the more schooled audience the range of materials available for Spanish-speaking audiences rather than used as the primary teaching tool for these different Latino audiences. Knowledge of the literacy level of the target audience in situations such as those just described is a must. Another illustration might further clarify the issues at hand relative to literacy.

Literacy and Cognitive Assessment Distortion

The interference of literacy with cultural factors in the appropriate evaluation of dementing illness can perhaps most clearly be seen in the area of cognitive assessment. As is known, the identification of Alzheimer's disease and of some related dementing conditions in their early stages is especially problematic because the symptoms, especially Alzheimer's disease, emerge in such an insidious manner as to be confused with other problems that also bring memory and orientation difficulties. For example, depression, medication misuse, and other physical illnesses present many of the same symptoms. To pinpoint some of the cognitive problems being encountered, the professional or provider will quite likely use some form of screening instrument to assess the client's or patient's cognitive capabilities. The most commonly used screen is the Mini-Mental Status Examination (MMSE; Folstein, Folstein, & McHough, 1975), or some derivative that can assess several key areas to encompass: (a) short-term memory capabilities, (b) orientation to time and place, (c) comprehension functions, and (d) attention and calculation skills.

From the start, the developers of the MMSE found that there were some educational effects in its application to the general population in that persons with less than 8 years of schooling generally do more poorly on the MMSE apart from any memory problems which exist (Anthony, Le Resche, Naiz, von Koroff, & Folstein, 1982). These findings have continued to be noted through the present (Mungas, 1996; Mungas, Marshall, Weldon, Haan, & Reed, 1996; Stern et al., 1992; Tombaugh & McIntyre, 1992). Other researchers also have noted educational effects with regard to specific ethnic groups, such as Hispanics (Bird, Canino, & Shrout, 1987; Escobar et al., 1986;

Lopez & Taussig, 1991) and African Americans (Holzer, Tischer, Leaf, & Myers, 1984; Holzer et al., 1986; Murden, McRae, Kaner, & Buckman, 1991). Similar problems have been noted with other populations around the world, such as the Chinese (Borrini, Dall'Ora, Della Sala, Marinelli, & Spinnler, 1989; Hill, Klauber, Salmon, Yu, Liu, Zhang, & Katzman, 1993; Katzman et al., 1988; LeCours et al., 1987; Li et al., 1989; Ogunniyi, Lekwauwa, & Osuntokun, 1991; Yu et al., 1989), the Thai (Phanthumchinda, Jitapunkul, Sitthi-Amorn, & Bunnag, 1991), and the Dutch (van der Cammen & van Harskamp, 1992). Paniagua (1994) speaks strongly to the point of avoiding biased instruments in making assessments, with the biases including lack of attention to the sociodemographic characteristics of the ethnocultural individual being evaluated. The central concern is that even if the evaluative tools are made culture fair, that is, transculturated into the appropriate cultural and linguistic idiom, education and literacy factors may still get in the way of a proper assessment (Helms, 1992; Valle, 1994).

Avoiding Literacy Stereotypes

At the same time, as with all other aspects of cross-cultural work, stereotypes must be avoided in the area of making literacy assessments. For example, as noted earlier, it must be recalled that some ethnocultural groups have literacy traditions that antedate those of Europe. Still others come from backgrounds that are based more on oral history. The first-generation Hmong people from Southeast Asia is an example of this category. Others, such as Latinos/Hispanic ethnic groups, present quite mixed profiles. In reality the picture with regard to the literacy issue is much more of a mixed variety, that is, a priori assumptions cannot be made with regard to any ethnically diverse group. A caregiver coming from a more literate culture may not be formally schooled, whereas another coming from a culture that emphasizes oral tradition may in fact be quite schooled.

TECHNIQUES FOR SORTING FACTORS
CONFUSED WITH CULTURE

Admittedly, at the point of direct contact with ethnically diverse clients it can be difficult to distinguish immediately if an attitude or behavior has its roots in the cultural or the social status (socioeconomic) domain. Even more seasoned intercultural engagement practitioners can experience such uncertainty. There are times, therefore, when developing appropriate distinctions can rest on some relatively pragmatic steps.

1. **The literature on ethnically diverse populations has to be read carefully.** For example, are the authors talking about poor people who happen to be of a specific ethnic group? Are they talking about literacy in general, or about literacy levels relative to a particular group? Regardless of the format within which the information is presented, in writings in conferences or in the media, it has to be examined for overgeneralizations and stereotypes about the group based on sociodemographic data.

2. **Learn to recognize the residual—that is, the long-enduring—effects of the factors of lower socioeconomic status, discrimination, and a lack of literacy.** The opportunity levels are different for many members of the society, especially with regard to ethnically diverse group members. The systems-coping demands of a highly technological environment such as that of the United States require much advance educationally and experientially based information and preparation. The society's institutional arrangements affect many ethnic groups differentially (Farley, 1995). As delineated in the Harris case (Case 7.2), the residual effects of racism, not culture, compounded the difficulties being experienced by the elder Mrs. Harris as well as by all concerned.

3. **Develop the ability to distinguish between social status and cultural factors in ethnically diverse interventions.** By doing so, the professional or provider can thereby make appropriate differentiations. As indicated in Case 7.1, not all ethnically diverse low-income people like to eat the same foods. Not all speak the same languages. Nor, for that matter, do they have the same historical past within the host society. These and other differences between groups can assist in avoiding the use of the discredited "culture-of-poverty" type analyses.

4. **Learn to work with the social status factors alongside the cultural framework.** Once properly sorted, the factors arising from the different domains can be blended within the overall acculturation continuum framework, as suggested in Chapter 2 (see Figure 2.3).

END NOTE: IS IT REALLY CULTURE, OR IS IT SOMETHING ELSE?

Researchers and practitioners alike report the willingness of ethnic minority caregivers and their elderly to engage with more formalized forms of services, including caregiving support groups within the area of Alzheimer's disease and related disorders. Segal and Wykle (1988–1989), Wood and Parham (1990), and Wykle and Segal (1991) note these responses on the part of African Americans; Taussig & Trejo (1992) does likewise with reference to Hispanics, as do Henderson (1992) and Henderson et al. (1993) as well as Cox and Monk (1990, 1993) with regard to both Hispanics and African American groups. Valle et al. (1989) highlight the service interaction activity of a mix of ethnocultural groups. These findings begin to address the cultural side of the service involvement and intercultural engagement process.

At the same time, professionals and providers have to broaden their approaches to be certain that several important factors do not bias their cultural assessments. Considerable harm can be done to the intercultural engagement process if ethnically diverse clients are assessed simply as low-income individuals to the exclusion of the ethnocultural dimension of their lives. The same can happen if such clients are relegated to the category of being only the victims of discrimination, or being nonliterate, or being part of a powerless ethnocultural group. These circumstances may be present; however, the intercultural assessment methodology asks the practitioner to examine all the facets of the ethnically diverse clients' lives to formulate the complete picture of the family's response to dementing illness. Professionals and providers can have confidence that, if care is taken to address both the cultural and social status facets of their clients' circumstances, appropriate cultural mapping assessments can be made. To this end, the professional or provider must, therefore, not only become sufficiently skilled to sort the different sets of factors but also determine where the overlap between culture and social status occurs within a single intercultural engagement situation (Miner, 1995).

Part Two

Integration of Cultural Mapping Concepts

Part Two presents an overview of the knowledge and skills required by the practitioner to appropriately implement the intercultural engagement/cultural mapping process. The content is a summary of the approach detailed in Part One. This shortened summary of the key concepts in the model is provided in an encapsulated format to facilitate the practitioner's ready access to the cultural mapping process.

Intercultural practice has a strong theoretical basis, but its overall strength comes from the actual application of the concepts. The ethnically diverse client group will be looking for professionals and providers who demonstrate an ability to carry the intercultural engagement effort directly to them. Conceptual understanding must be illustrated to the ethnically diverse client through the actual meeting of the patient's and the family members' needs. As most practitioners know, the measure of one's interventive capabilities comes from being able to implement concepts learned sequentially, in a holistic manner. Interventive competence is also demonstrated by the practitioner's ability to appropriately draw on theory to meet the demands of the immediate interventive situation.

Chapter 8 examines a number of professional and provider capabilities that can be carried over from general practice to culturally focused interventions. For example, *active listening* is promoted in most practitioner training programs. In intercultural practice, this practice skill has to be converted into being able to listen with one's *cultural ear* carefully attuned to the ethnically diverse client group's needs and concerned in the context of the group's linguistic, interactional, and value orientations.

The principle of being conscious of one's own values, and not imposing them on the client, is likewise inculcated within many professional and provider training programs. This orientation can be readily converted into the intercultural engagement principle of restraining one's own cultural and/or professional beliefs while permitting the ethnically diverse client's normative expectations to come forward first within the cultural mapping process. In addition, practitioners must remain alert to their tendency to rely primarily on technical insights and professional jargon to explain dementing illness and attendant careplans to an ethnically diverse clientele. What is required, therefore, is that practitioners convert what are often promoted as standard practice principles into culturally compatible formats. The chapter provides guidelines for the professional or provider to achieve this desired outcome.

Chapter 9 brings all of the pieces of the cultural mapping model together. The chapter walks the practitioner through the various steps in the cultural assessment process to include the key considerations that go into implementing a culturally attuned careplan. The reader may find some redundancy with earlier chapters; however, the intent is to assist the professional or provider to see the model in a broad context. The earlier chapter-by-chapter discussion in Part One was aimed at elaborating the different stages and the subsequent steps involved in the cultural mapping process. The aim of Chapter 9 is to pull the intercultural engagement framework together.

Cultural mapping and the problem-solving methods of the various helping professions go hand in hand with regard to meeting the dementia-care needs of ethnically diverse populations. As envisioned here, cultural mapping allows professionals and providers to fine tune their interventive strategies for application to ethnoculturally distinct situations. To this end a specific formula, the LEARN problem-solving strategy, is discussed as an adjunct to the overall intercultural engagement effort. The special feature of the LEARN technique is that it enables the cross-cultural practitioner to model the problem-solving process for ethnically diverse client groups whose members may be less familiar with the "cultural" features of dementia-care systems.

Linking the cultural mapping approach to problem solving enriches both. When used together, the practitioner can assess not only the clients' dementia-care needs but also the cultural dimensions of the situation. Moreover, both approaches are necessary to appropriately serve family members and individuals who linguistically and culturally belong to groups outside the mainstream English-speaking resource system. Basically, the comprehensive approach can be fashioned into a tool for extending existing services to currently undeserved populations that are nonetheless confronting dementing illness.

An added feature of Part Two is the cultural mapping/cultural assessment checklist in Chapter 9, which offers the practitioner a quick but comprehensive overview of the full cultural mapping process. In this manner, professionals and providers, as well as their parent organizations, can identify key areas on which to concentrate while searching elsewhere through Part One for an in-depth elaboration of specific concepts. In addition, the Part Two review, which appears somewhat midstream in the text, allows for a transition to Part Three, which looks beyond the direct client engagement processes to the responsibilities of the dementia-care organization as a whole in supporting the intercultural engagement process.

Chapter 8

Special Professional and Provider Preparation

Many professional and provider training programs for health and human services personnel teach *active listening skills* (J. Anderson, 1997; Hepworth & Larsen, 1993; Ivey, 1994; Schneider-Corey & Corey, 1992; Zastrow, 1985). The content covered may focus on establishing clinician–patient rapport, on maintaining administrator–employee working relationships, or on reinforcing the organization's market linkages. At their core, the listening principles promote a consumer-centered emphasis, and it is this emphasis that can form the basis of turning general active listening capabilities into *cultural listening* capabilities (Brislin & Yoshida, 1994; Brownlee, 1978; Gudykunst, 1994; Harris & Moran, 1987).

This part of the text builds on these generic listening skills, which, when properly tailored to the cultural situation, enable the professional and provider to engage culturally diverse populations. The focus will be on: (a) augmenting active cross-cultural listening skills, (b) fine-tuning this capability into nonjudgmental listening, (c) blocking the imposition of the professional's or provider's culture into the intercultural engagement situation, (d) guarding against the tendency to use technical jargon in cross-ethnic communications, and (e) maintaining attention to the literacy level of the ethnically diverse lay audience clientele when engaged in intercultural communication. These skills can be subsumed under the concept of *multicultural empathy* suggested by Ridley & Lingle (1996).

From an overall perspective, listening skills can be considered a core skill expected of the professional or provider. However, from the intercultural engagement viewpoint, these skills need to be examined for the possibility of the presence of ethnocentrism. In this instance the ethnocentrism will be coming from the practitioner's own service culture. If professionals or providers are not on guard, their own service-culture value orientations can seep into the intercultural engagement situation, thereby impeding the cultural mapping/intercultural exchange process.

CROSS-CULTURAL ACTIVE LISTENING

Cross-cultural active listening—what Ivey (1994, p. 13) calls "the basic listening sequence"—whether conducted directly by a bilingual professional or provider or by a bicultural-pair, is the doorway to the understanding of a host of culture-specific caregiving contexts. Most important, it can lead to insights about how (a) the caregiver actually sees the responsibility of providing the required daily care, (b) the caregiver and the family/significant others look at their joint responsibilities with respect to the care of the dementia-affected elder, and (c) the caregiver and the significant other family members play out their roles within the context of their overall ethnic group value orientations. Furthermore, interculturally active listening leads to an awareness of any *cultural contradictions* that may be present in the care situation relative to the caregiver's traditional normative expectations about how the other family members are responding to the situation with regard to their different levels of acculturation.

In this context the professional's or provider's alertness can be heightened so that he or she can identify behaviors or attitudes that may reflect the ethnic client's *cultural paralysis;* that is, through cross-cultural active listening the professional or provider can often identify whether the caregiver is simply being noncompliant or is immobilized because he or she is caught between traditional beliefs and the suggested actions coming from the health or human service system.

> Case 8.1a. Mrs. Herrera, who was being cared for at home, had entered the last stages of her Alzheimer's disease concurrent with having just recovered from a respiratory disorder. At the family's insistence, and with the family physician's agreement, she had been returned home for her aftercare, which required both the use of oxygen and tube feeding. However, the physician felt he needed clarification about future care and what to do if resuscitation were necessary. The family seemed divided on the issue. Home health care had been prescribed for the first 8 weeks, and a nurse from the home health care agency had been assigned the case. Being a monolingual English-speaker herself, the nurse first spoke to the monolingual Spanish-speaking family members through the younger bilingual daughter, who served as the family go-between with providers. The bilingual daughter indicated that she favored a do-not-resuscitate order, but she said that the family needed time to discuss the issues involved. The nurse noted that the eldest daughter, the primary caregiver, did not respond at all to any of the translated discussion. She decided it was important to postpone any further considerations until she could team up with the agency's bilingual aide.

Application of her own professional listening skills enabled the nurse to recognize that something was blocking the discussion of the resuscitation concerns but, not being bilingual/bicultural, she could not tell exactly what. She also was uncomfortable having to rely totally on the bilingual younger daughter. From the onset of her involvement, she had felt the need to pair up with the agency's bilingual aide but could not because of a scheduling conflict. At the same time she was required by her parent organization to conduct a home care health status check as soon as possible after Mrs. Herrera's discharge. As she thought back over the session she felt it might have been better just to check the patient and not to engage in the discussion of the resuscitation issue, especially through the family translator.

> Case 8.1b. The bicultural-pair returned a week later, and a family conference took place after the nurse had checked on Mrs. Herrera's condition. On starting, both the nurse and the bilingual aide felt considerable tension. The bilingual daughter, usually quite a verbal and outgoing person, stayed mostly in the background. The primary caregiver herself, the eldest daughter, did not come into the group discussion at all but stayed in the bedroom caring for Mrs. Herrera. The other family members present took the information in Spanish that was handed out but made few comments. The conversation was at times quite disjointed because of the comings and goings of various family members. Realizing that the conference was not really going anywhere, the bilingual aide indicated that he wanted to greet the patient. As he came into the bedroom, he noted that the caregiver, sitting by her mother, did not look up at him but rather continued to attend to her mother. At no point did the caregiver talk directly about anything pertaining to the prolonging-life-support issues. Rather she profusely began to express her thanks to the agency and the doctors for all they had done and asked the aide to convey her gratitude to the agency.

The aide recognized the form of *cultural dismissal* that had taken place. In Spanish, the resuscitation discussion was an *asunto cerrado* (a closed matter). On exiting, the bicultural-pair complimented the family on how they were caring for Mrs. Herrera. As the aide and the nurse were getting into their respective cars, the aide told the nurse that the family's indecision was, in effect, a decision.

All such situations like those just described in Cases 8.1a and 8.1b are much more complex than the narration indicates. However, it was clear that, although the nurse was not Spanish-speaking, her initial recognition of family tension in regard to the resuscitation concerns were on target. The pattern was confirmed the following week. It was evident that even the bilingual daughter, who had personally accepted the resuscitation issue, was deferring to the more traditionally oriented family members. It can often happen that traditional culture will dictate the actions to be taken; in the Herrera case, no action on the resuscitation question became in essence a family decision. Although the professional or provider, including the bicultural-pair, may have seen a do-not-resuscite order as a more effective way to proceed, the family's views had to be respected.

In these instances, cross-cultural active listening enables the practitioner to see that, no matter how seemingly "good" or "rational" the formal service plans may appear, the *cultural signals* that are being communicated cannot be ignored. If they are, the suggested plan of action, notwithstanding its strong merit, stands a strong chance of becoming stuck. Basically, the technique of being alert to the ethnic group members' affective and behavioral signals allows the practitioner to work closer in harmony with the group's own cultural norms.

NONJUDGMENTAL "ACTIVE" LISTENING

There is a further application of the technique of cross-cultural active listening that could be termed *nonjudgmental listening* (Harris & Moran, 1987, p. 95; Meyerson, 1994). This enhanced approach takes the notion of active listening a step further into the cultural core of the ethnically diverse target client group. The approach allows the professional or provider to really enter the perceptual world of the cultural group. From a cultural practice perspective, the nonjudgmental aspect of the active-listening technique enables the target ethnic group members to freely express their indigenous understanding about dementing illness without the inhibitions that accompany the family members' contacts with professional and providers, particularly if the family members are under the impression that the practitioners will be making comments and corrections to their views.

> Case 8.2. The needs of the Fredrico's (a Chamorro family recently arrived from Guam), had been brought to the attention of the clinic staff member. The eldest son, a career civilian employee of the Navy, had been reassigned to the mainland for a period of 3 years. Along with his wife and 2 teenage daughters, he felt it was important to bring his mother, a *latico-bodig* dementia-affected elder. *Latico-bodig* is a dual Alzheimer's/ Parkinson's disease condition which is prevalent among the native Chamorro people of Guam. It was clear to the clinic professional that the caregiving daughter-in-law was overwhelmed. Also, the relocation from the Island of Guam, a U.S. territory, had generated culture shock. The clinic practitioner brought up the possibility of in-home supportive services for which a family was eligible. This suggestion generated considerable turmoil within the family. The son spoke about his belief that it was the family's traditional responsibility to care for the mother. He indicated that among the Chamorro people there was a belief that such illness as *latico-bodig* demonstrated a lack of harmony with the island gods and that this situation would be best balanced if the family did the caring. He said that although he understood the actual medical nature of the dementing condition, he felt that many family members in Guam would be quite concerned if family obligations and traditions were not observed. Fortunately, there was a way through the difficulties. Although at first taken aback by the rationale given by the son, the practitioner said nothing. Instead, the practitioner suggested an alternative arrangement wherein in-home support hours could be paid to the teenage granddaughters who divided the responsibilities between themselves, thereby accommodating their customs.

Before the initial home visit, the Alzheimer's clinic professional had read about the *latico-bodig* condition, which affects the Chamorro people. However, she was not fully versed in the native Guamanian beliefs. Although they were new to her, she nonetheless acted in a nonjudgmental manner. The fact that the professional's cultural ear was properly tuned in to listen to the nuances of what the Chamorro family members were saying introduced flexibility into the situation, allowing for an accommodation to be made. The nonjudgmental active-listening technique often goes a long way toward the resolution of what on the surface may appear to be insoluble problems between the ethnic group members and the practitioner's beliefs and value orientations.

ENGAGING IN CULTURALLY APPROPRIATE COMMUNICATION

Active listening also brings with it an awareness of the importance of being versed in the native language of the target ethnic group members and, in the absence of this capability, of the need to be able to link up with native speakers from the ethnic group. Over and above the interest of observing cultural proprieties, professionals and providers have to be certain that the communications about the disease aspects of the dementing illness are conveyed to even the most monolingual non-English-speaking members of the ethnic client group.

Admittedly, the demand to be able to communicate in the target ethnic group's native language can create some pressures for practitioners. It is obvious that no individual professional or provider, or even a total service organization, can possibly cover all of the ethnic group languages potentially active in their respective service regions. Nor can they always find sufficient bilingual/bicultural candidates with whom to form bicultural-pairs. This is especially true in major metropolitan areas, where there may be 50 or more languages or dialects in active daily use. It is equally obvious that ethnically diverse family members, particularly those closest to their native language, cannot be expected to communicate only in English and that an understanding about dementia will not be communicated if only English is used. In a like manner, in the absence of such a bicultural capability on the part of the practitioner, care has to be taken not to put the bilingual family member, who becomes the go-between, into a situation where there is a conflict of interest between the agency's and the family's interests. Above all, the needs of the dementia-affected elder cannot be put aside indefinitely, until the appropriate bicultural resources are found. There are times when action must be taken.

> Case 8.3. Mr. Assad, a Chaldean immigrant, his brother, and their wives and children had resettled on the West coast from Chicago. The remaining family, two sisters and several female cousins, had stayed in the East. The eldest son now found himself in a quandary. Their mother's Alzheimer's disease had progressed to the point that she could no longer be left alone either in their homes or with the relatives back in Chicago. No single household could provide full-time care at home. This put a special strain on the female blood kin who, by tradition, were expected to care for the mother. The daughters-in-law in turn were upset that their husbands' status in the community would be diminished if that tradition were not upheld.
>
> Mr. Assad called a multicultural outreach dementia service for help. After careful assessment, the culturally sensitive, but non-Chaldean, practitioner located a day care center that was an annex of a skilled-nursing facility in Chicago with Aramaic-speaking staff and residents. She suggested that Mr. Assad talk to all of the family about exploring this alternative, not forgetting to stress that the female family members had to visit the setting and agree that using it would be in concert with their culture's expectations about family caregiving.

The eldest son served as the family spokesperson and go-between. In the end, a family consensus was reached that the day center enrollment in Chicago would be initiated. The practitioner, however, was never sure if all of the family members fully understood dementia, even after all of her explanations to Mr. Assad. However, it did appear that everyone understood that the elder Mrs. Assad would get better care in the Chicago program and that the family traditions would be upheld.

The provider from the multicultural outreach program involved in Case 8.3 had come prepared. She had brought along some visual materials on Alzheimer's disease. During part of the meeting she had Mr. Assad translate an explanation of the physical nature of Alzheimer's disease. She had also obtained a brochure from the prospective placement agency, with some of the description in Aramaic. It was not a perfect session with regard to full assurance that everyone understood the rationale for placement. However, the family members present did agree to check out the day care program, and the solution was not imposed from outside but rather emerged from the circumstances in which the family members now found themselves.

It was said in Chapter 5 that it is "best" not to use family members as the bicultural communicators as they may be placed in a conflicted position. It has also been suggested that, if one is not conversant in the target ethnic group's language, it is "best" to pair up with a bilingual intercultural communicator from the community. Given the circumstances facing the practitioner in Case 8.3, neither of these suggestions could be observed. In such situations, therefore, the "best" approach is to respond in a culturally appropriate manner to the requests from the family. If the multicultural outreach program provider had come to the family with the idea of initiating a placement, quite a different outcome might have occurred.

ADDITIONAL PRACTITIONER-PREPAREDNESS CONSIDERATIONS

Active listening also includes attention to the literacy level of the client group. As indicated in Chapter 4, case 4.2, the professional or practitioner has to be careful not to send messages that go over the heads of the ethnic group members even when the intercultural communications are conducted in the native language of the intended audience. As indicated, even bilingual/bicultural professionals must guard against imparting information that is overly complex or that takes considerable effort to be integrated by the ethnically diverse client, particularly where low levels of schooling are involved.

Case 8.4. Mr. Yepes, a Mexican-heritage Latino, had originally come to the Bilingual Alzheimer's Clinic a year previously, when his wife had been diagnosed with Alzheimer's disease. He and his wife, now in their 70s, had spent the greater part of their lives as agricultural field workers. The clinic had been able to serve this monolingual Spanish-speaking family and had provided videos as well as printed information about Alzheimer's disease, along with an in-depth exit conference. In the midst of the clinic's annual review conference with the neurologist, Mr. Yepes spontaneously turned and asked *"?Por que la llamaron la enfermedad de Alzheimer?"* ("Why did they call it Alzheimer's disease?").

The practitioner's explanation that the disease had been named after its discoverer, a German physician, cleared up a minor but nonetheless troublesome concern that the caregiver had been reluctant to bring up—even though he had been provided material in Spanish that dealt with this same point. His concerns could perhaps have been handled from the start if the practitioners had been extra attentive and not assumed that handing over the written material and subsequent frequent naming of the disorder was sufficient. However, even with earlier inputs such questions are not unexpected, particularly from individuals whose previous experience has been away from the more scientific and schooled aspects of daily living.

It is important to use the target ethnic group's native language. At the same time the cross-cultural active-listening approach indicates that the practitioner needs to check and recheck that the technical and medical sides of the dementing illness message has been internalized. If this step is missing, there is a very strong chance that the members of the target ethnic audience will miss large pieces of the intended communication.

PRACTITIONER'S CULTURE: POSSIBLE BRIDGES

As has been noted, professionals and providers come from strong service-focused cultures that have their own formal languages, their ways of interacting with the client and the public, and defined value orientations relative to how the service exchanges between the client and the practitioner should be conducted (Brownlee, 1978; Stein, 1990). Professionals and providers are likewise infused with the mainstream U.S. host society's cultural values, although they are not always consciously aware of carrying them around. Therefore, if the practitioner lacks self-awareness of these influences, this can definitely get in the way of accommodating the ethnically diverse client's world. Moreover, as has been indicated, even ethnically diverse bilingual/bicultural providers can fail to take into account the impact of their own professional culture when dealing with members of their own ethnic group. However, it takes only the experience of engaging in communication with the ethnic community residents for bilingual/bicultural practitioners to be confronted with the reality of how "professionalized" and "Americanized" they have become when communicating with and engaging others closer to his or her own culture of origin.

> Case 8.5. The Alzheimer's-disease-and-related-disorders community educator had just shown the Vietnamese-language "Orientation to Alzheimer's Disease" video to the assembled members of the Asian Pacific Senior Center. He was responding to a question of just how the brain becomes impaired and stopped himself in midsentence. He realized that, although he was speaking Vietnamese, he was still using terms such as *the hippocampus, the cortex,* and *damage to neuronal tissue*. He realized quickly that he had clearly lost the audience. Reversing gears, he drew an analogy for his audience of how the brain's network for communication could be compared to having all the electrical cords in one's house deteriorate and break off connections from one another. Certainly, this approach would not be considered technically sound in the classroom or at a health provider meeting, but it began to get the point across to the particular audience in attendance.

Aside from the high technical level at which professionals and providers may approach communications, as in Case 8.5, there are other impediments that can emerge between practitioners and their ethnically diverse clients. One such impediment is the potential conflict of perspective, discussed in Chapter 4, between the *cultural engagement style* desired by many ethnically diverse groups and the *getting-to-the-point* approach often preferred by professionals or providers, or at least their parent organizations (Tempo & Saito, 1996). A similar barrier can come up around the ethnically diverse client's need to maintain affectively appropriate intercultural engagement customs according to which pleasantries are exchanged for a period of time and the more objective interactive styles generally taught to and followed by professionals and providers. In this context, the professionals or providers can give the impression that they are distancing themselves from the contact. However, what is really happening is that the practitioners are following their training, which teaches them not to impose their feelings on the client. All of this may not be understood by the ethnically diverse client group members who may be expecting to see a reflection of their own interpersonal engagement styles.

On looking at the matter more closely, the contradictions between the practitioner's expectations and ethnoculturally based interactional expectations may be more apparent than real. For example, when practitioners follow the rules for establishing relationships within a specific ethnocultural group, they are really following the principles taught in many professional programs as to "starting where the client is." When practitioners engage in retrospection about the possible impact of their own professionalism on the client group they are only applying the principle of "conscious use of self." When an ethnically diverse family presents the practitioner with a solution to a dementing illness care problem that is different than planned, but feasible to themselves, professionals and providers are allowing for "client self-determination." If looked at in this light, the rules of intercultural engagement often only broaden the application of the principles noted, even though they might have first been conceptualized for mainstream English-speaking cultural populations.

All in all, adopting some of the target ethnic group's cultural exchange rituals does not preclude the application of professional objectivity with regard to providing assessment and careplanning assistance to ethnically diverse dementia-affected elders and their family members; rather, there are a number of "client engagement and empowerment" principles, espoused by the major helping professions engaged in dementia-service, that can be put to work. For example, many professional disciplines espouse the principle that the "client, and not the practitioner, must *own* the solution to the problem." Also, in the area of self-image development, clients are encouraged "to accept their own strengths" or "to see the positives in themselves." These and other approaches can be modified to fit the cultural situation that the dementia-care practitioner encounters.

In seeking further to enhance the intercultural exchange process, the professional or provider can proceed by actively using the Intercultural communication model (see Figure 4.1). Through this process, the practitioner can track how important messages related to dementing illness are getting through. If such communications do not initially take hold, such as in the Yepes caregiving situation (Case 8.4), the professional or provider can remedy the situation at a later date. Additionally, by taking the necessary time and making an effort to follow the expected rules for cultural rapport, professionals and providers are actually establishing the kinds of client–practitioner mutual trust ties that are preferred for helping families over the long course of a dementing illness. Finally, the effort expended toward reducing the impact of the practitioner's own culture facilitates the earlier surfacing of the ethnically diverse family's own help-seeking and help-accepting expectations and approaches, which are needed before the dementia-careplan can be put into place.

Using, But Not Imposing, Technical Jargon

A balance must be maintained in communications about dementing illness to ethnically diverse client group members. The professional or practitioner cannot always "water down" the technical language or use substitute analogies in every instance. There are sound reasons for using and maintaining the technical language surrounding dementing illness. For example, the design of careplans with ethnically diverse populations often involves attention to technical details with respect to eligibility, billing, and other forms that need to be completed to maintain coverage for services performed. The specific diagnosis of possible or probable Alzheimer's disease, or the presence of multi-infarct dementia or any other dementing condition, needs to be explicitly identified for follow-up interventive purposes and, as has been noted earlier, there are no intercultural substitutes for the terms *Alzheimer's, Pick's,* or *Huntington's chorea,* or any of the other specifically designated dementing conditions, which bear the names of their original discoverers.

Therefore, regardless of whether individual professionals or providers might prefer other approaches, patients and their family members must use this formal language for certain situations related to obtaining the best service possible for their dementia-affected family member. The issues apply to the many different aspects of the dementing illness service continuum, whether they be legal, fiscal, or social in scope. The agencies involved will need the information processed in their language. Here the bilingual/bicultural professional or provider, or the bicultural-pair, must bridge back from the indigenous cultural understandings to be sure that the required forms and information are provided so as to ensure the flow of services to the elder in need. In these circumstances it is still incumbent on the professional or provider to assure that the members of the ethnically diverse client group understand what is occurring and what is meant by the different process and forms. This activity is particularly needed when the ethnic group members may lack sufficient background to initially grasp the formal medical, health, or other service system terminology being used (Brownlee, 1978: Chapter 3).

STEPS TO ENSURE CROSS-CULTURAL ACTIVE LISTENING

Professionals and providers can consider a number of working principles to help ensure that they are indeed prepared for intercultural engagement and communication.

1. **Practitioners need to adopt a posture that is culturally attuned to the contacts and communications they intend to make.** This implies that pro-

fessionals and providers are able to extend the concept of active listening to encompass multiple cultural situations, none of which may be the same. This also implies that the professional or provider restrain the impulse to quickly arrive at conclusions that may be ethnocentric in focus, that is, conclusions that are driven forward by the professional's or the provider's own culture rather than the ethnically diverse client's. Basically, the practitioner must not only actively listen across cultures but also behave in a nonjudgmental manner, especially in the context of dementing illness, which brings with it so many stressors to the patient and the family.

2. **Practitioners can make links to many of the practice and intervention principles that operate in their respective disciplines.** Connections can be made between practice principles from the professional's or provider's training background and the ethnically diverse client's world. These include such concepts as "beginning the intervention and moving it at the client's pace" and "assuring that the client owns the change process being initiated." There are many other broad principles, discussed above, that emerge from the various professional and provider disciplines engaged in dementia care. These principles also need to be examined for their cross-cultural import. The practitioner's task is to directly examine how any working principle can be extended to the ethnocultural client's value and normative outlooks. As noted earlier, forcing the ethnically diverse client into the professional practice frameworks as they stand in their original format is interculturally inappropriate. It may appear difficult at first to recast approaches that have been developed for mainstream cultural populations, but with practice the transculturation strategy becomes easier and provides an overall better mesh with the client's situational realities and native cultural expectations. One does not become less professional in a cross-cultural context; rather, professionalism is enhanced through adaptation of core skills and orientations to the demands of the multicultural dementia-care environment. Seasoned professionals and providers recognize the value of this approach (Aranda, 1990; Ridley & Lingle, 1996).

3. **Practitioners need to be clear as to when to use and not to use technical/ professional/health and service system jargon.** The technical languages surrounding dementia care, however essential, can at times get in the way of working with ethnically diverse families such as getting them connected to services and/or clarifying how to meet eligibility criteria. The "jargon" that is used withing the different fields actually arises in a cultural milieu. These service languages can include the seemingly endless acronyms used to identify different types of needs or services. For example, the use of acronyms such as ADLs and IADLs with ethnically diverse clients who rely on their native languages can confuse the discussion. It is better for the professional or provider to indicate specific activities of daily living and instrumental activities of daily living in the intercultural exchange with the client. From an overall perspective, decisions about when to use or not to use jargon can be more appropriately handled if the jargon is viewed in a cultural context. It is one more language that requires intercultural bridging.

END NOTE

Professionals and providers have to recognize the potential impact of both their personal cultural orientations and their service culture on the proposed intercultural engagement situation. Active listening and engaging implies an ongoing conscious awareness of what one is doing and saying as well as of what the client says and does. These processes imply a capability on the part of the practitioner to blend both streams of information into a culturally coherent interventive approach. The most appropriate measure of readiness for intercultural practice is when professionals or providers have internalized the cultural mapping approach as a normal component of their everyday client engagement methodology. In this regard the practitioner will have reached what Gudykunst (1994, pp. 5–6) calls a state of *unconscious competence,* that is, the professionals or providers have now honed their intercultural engagement skills into a "practice art" built on observing sound cross-cultural methodological principles for intergroup interaction.

Chapter 9

Cultural Mapping Process: A Summary

The points to be covered are summarized in Box 9.1: A Cultural Mapping/Intercultural Assessment Checklist. For beginners in the intercultural engagement arena, it might be helpful to maintain a cultural engagement checklist for use as either the face-to-face or telephone contact takes place. The more experienced intercultural engagement practitioners will have internalized some form of checklist into their working repertoire. This is performed in much the same manner as the experienced professional or provider does when incorporating new features of intake or assessment protocols relative to the complexities of dementing illness symptomatology. The checklist basically parallels the cultural mapping/intercultural assessment process as discussed throughout Part One.

CULTURAL ASSESSMENT STARTING POINTS

The cultural mapping process actually begins before the first face-to-face contact with the ethnically diverse client group members seeking assistance for their dementia-affected family member. For example, the bicultural practitioner or provider, or the bicultural-pair, can begin to assemble information about the ethnically diverse population that is being targeted for dementia-related contact or services. The biculturality of the practitioner does not preclude updating one's knowledge of the current status and

1. **Ethnicity/Acculturation**
  a. Caller's/contact's culture-of-
    origin/ethnicity
  b. Patient's/family members' culture
    of origin/ethnicity
	THE ACCULTURATION CONTINUUM
	FORMULATION IS APPLIED

2. **History/Background** Cultural/historical past/present background notes/content	THE FAMILY'S/ETHNIC GROUP'S CULTURAL HISTORY IS MAPPED

3. **Language**
  a. Caller's/contact's language preference
  b. Family constellation language
    preferences (note all key members)
	THE FAMILY'S LINGUISTIC
	PREFERENCES ARE IDENTIFIED

4. **Relationships** The family's/significant others' relationships, both positive/negative along with decision-influencing patterns, etc.	THE FAMILY CONSTELLATION IS MAPPED; ECO MAPPING CAN BE USED
5. **Values/Beliefs** Value/belief orientations to include nuances and mixes of orientations; also the indigenous cultural under- standing of dementing illness	VALUES/BELIEFS/NORMATIVE EXPECTATIONS ARE IDENTIFIED
6. **Cultural Confounds** Social status issues/concerns that might distort the cultural assessment	FACTORS APART FROM CULTURE ARE NOTED/INCORPORATED

Box 9.1 Cultural mapping/intercultural assessment checklist.

the cultural–historical presence of the ethnic group members within the local community. Additional refinements to prior knowledge are always useful, especially when
local factors, such as a large influx of new members of the ethnic group, take place,
or community tensions become heightened, or any number of current events occur
that have impact on the ethnic group members' lives. Moreover, the collection of
additional pertinent information is a corollary to the standard procedure used by most
professionals or providers who consistently add to their community information resources on an ongoing basis.

In essence, the professional or provider begins the intercultural engagement process at Step 2 of the Cultural Mapping Checklist, *History/Background* of the ethnic
group. However, the content is assembled in such a manner as to address the issues
highlighted in Step 1, the application of the acculturation continuum formulation. As
the reader will recall, in using the acculturation continuum model, the practitioner
identifies linguistic–communicational, interactional, and value–belief system behaviors that assist in identifying the ethnically diverse client group members within the
members' ethnocultural context. The model likewise assists the professional or provider to sort out social status factors, such as income and literacy levels, which are
often incorrectly mixed in with the cultural analysis being made. In point of fact,

practitioners need to see Step 1 as permeating all aspects of the implementation of the cultural mapping process.

Direct Contact

Direct contact with ethnically diverse clients can occur in any number of ways, just as with any other population: in person, in the community, in the clinic setting, over the telephone, or even by written correspondence. Regardless of the means of contact, the professional and provider must be ready to engage in culturally compatible ways. At the moment of intercultural contact, the professional or provider must be tactful. One does not engage in a series of questions about the contact person's cultural background. Reiterating what was indicated in Chapters 2 and 6, ethnic group members do not necessarily carry their cultural background in neat conceptual packages; rather, the practitioner focuses on the presenting problem in regard to the dementia-affected person's symptoms as well as the issues being raised by the contact person and/or family members. This feature does not change across cultures. The ethnically diverse clients will be calling or making contact about dementing illness concerns, not about their culture.

However, the assumption is that the professional or provider is already alert to cultural data gathering, because the process has already started in terms of the background preparatory work. From here, the practitioner immediately begins to listen with a third ear, in this case the *culturally attuned* third ear.

Ongoing Process

It should be clear from the onset that the checklist cannot be completed at the first contact, even by the most interculturally experienced practitioner. There are too many cultural variables to consider. Moreover, as has been suggested throughout the prior discussion, ethnically diverse families will tend to keep many aspects of their lives and preferences private and begin to indicate them only as the intercultural rapport deepens between the practitioner and the caregiver/family members. This should not deter the development of initial impressions in each of the six areas listed in the checklist.

Two practical actions can be taken at this initial phase of the cultural mapping/ intercultural assessment effort. First, the impressions received should be regarded only as assumptions relative to the cultural aspects of the ethnic group process. There is a likelihood that these early impressions will be modified as the contact deepens. As the professional's or provider's experience deepens, it can happen that many of the initial cultural mapping impressions will be confirmed within the later stages of the complete assessment. As more such impressions are eventually verified, practitioners can gauge the growth of their intercultural assessment capabilities. At the same time, even senior intercultural practitioners will experience the need to alter their perceptions of the target ethnic group's cultural processes as time passes.

Second, the checklist can also be used to track areas of cultural understanding that remain unclear or are missing at the initial phases of the intercultural contact process. Open questions can likewise be noted alongside the appropriate step on the checklist. Knowing what cultural information is still missing during the assessment and overall intercultural engagement process is in itself an important intercultural engagement skill. It relates to the practice principle that *defining* a given situation is also knowing what gaps in information exist.

Side Note: Importance of a Family History

Step 2 of the Cultural Mapping Checklist calls for more than an overview history of the ethnic group. From a dementia-care perspective, the professional or provider needs to acquire a much more detailed cultural–historical profile of the caregiving family members and the dementia-affected elder. In Case 6.5, the primary caregiver, Mrs. Morales, expected her children to have internalized her example and values with regard to caregiving. In her own upbringing one was always *culturally alert* and automatically watched the caring activities being played out. Assuming the caregiving role and its attendant responsibilities was therefore a natural and unspoken extension of the role modeling to which she had been exposed. Now she was replaying what her enculturated experience dictated, albeit under different environmental circumstances of life in the U.S. host society ambience. Mrs. Morales's children, however, had not made this internalization. For one, they had had a different enculturation, which required the external prodding of the practitioner for them to respond to the silent but deeply felt needs of their mother. All in all, knowing the cultural–historical background of the client is vitally important to the careplanning process.

> Case 9.1. Mrs. Cardenas had developed a great aversion to either the shower or the bathtub, actually becoming combative when entering either one. Hygienically, the situation was critical, as Mrs. Cardenas was also incontinent. Among the family information that had been gathered was the fact that as a girl the mother had bathed in a galvanized tin bathtub, with water occasionally added as needed by being poured over one's head. It was suggested that the caregiver try to replicate this situation. The caregiver obtained a sizable galvanized tub that would fit into the shower. When it came time to bathe her mother, she would call to her and bang the tub. The effort was rewarded when the mother's resistance to bathing stopped.

It appears that some connection had been made to the dementia-affected elder's childhood memories. This information, however, would not have been available without a thorough family cultural history. Although all aspects of the family's and the dementia-affected individual's past will not be pertinent in all instances, there will be times that the professional or provider can make practical use of such information.

THE LANGUAGE ARENA

Language issues, as related to ethnicity, surface at the point of contact. By means of the background information-gathering activity, the professional or provider will have determined the overall language capabilities of the ethnic group as a whole, for example, if the group members are primarily monolingual in their native language, bilingual, and so on. However, each family situation will bring its own linguistic preferences with it. There are no general rules as to what the professional or provider will find in each situation; therefore, the bilingual/bicultural practitioner or the bicultural-pair needs to be ready for any mix. Some ethnic client families will be monolingual in their own idiom. Others will be bilingual and, if an ethnic group resides in a host society such as that of the U.S., the practitioner should not be surprised to find that large portions of the family group members, including more of the second- or third-generation members, will be primarily English speakers, although a good portion of these will still retain their bilinguality. Again, this will vary from family to family and from group to group. However, with regard to the needs of the dementia-affected elder, who in most instances will relate to her or his native language, practitioners or bicultural-pairs must be proficient in this idiom so as to provide for a free and easy intercultural exchange.

As the practitioner–client relationship deepens, the professional or provider will find that the more medical and scientific aspects of the disease will be able to be communicated, even if the native language does not contain the terms. In the short run this is sometimes difficult; however, caregivers and family members/significant others, across cultures, generally have an interest in knowing as much as possible about what is affecting their family member. Here, though, the professional or provider needs to remain watchful about introducing too much complexity into the explanations, as discussed in Chapter 8 and below in Chapter 12. An approach that can be used is to leave printed materials with the family members who are most likely to respond to such content and allow the questions to emerge from the family group itself. If the practitioner has the opportunity to accompany the family to a diagnostic evaluation or to any other similar event, this can also be an excellent moment to introduce additional dementia-specific information. Professional or provider contacts with the family after their clinical appointments are equally productive. In this manner communications can be paced with the family members' growing understanding of the illness process.

All the while throughout the intercultural communication process the professional or provider will be well served by remaining alert to the application of the intercultural communication framework outlined in Figure 4.1. Language is the vehicle whereby individuals communicate their attitudes, feelings, and underlying normative views. These messages are encoded and decoded, properly or improperly throughout the communication process. This in turn is the reason why it is crucial that the practitioner either be bilingual/bicultural or be part of a bicultural-pair, with reference to the ethnic group being targeted for services. Much of what is cultural is contained in the nuances of the exchanges that take place between the communicators. As noted in Chapter 4, in the more traditionally oriented ethnic groups one can denote the different statuses between the communicators linguistically, with the senior or higher status individual receiving more deference and formal recognition than a peer or lower status person. These signals will be communicated not just in the salutations but also in the tone of voice and in the body language that accompanies an exchange.

A skilled bilingual/bicultural practitioner–communicator can begin to document this kind of information, adding to the cultural mapping information being assembled relative to the ethnically diverse client group. Without access to the ethnic group's language, the professional or provider is often left in the dark. It is true that the practitioner can make use of the family bilingual go-between. Many ethnically diverse families will have one or more members who can speak English, particularly when there are younger, second- and third-generation members. As with the Chaldean family (Case 8.3), there are times when the professional or provider has no choice but to make use of the family go-between.

However, several cautionary remarks need to be repeated here regarding the use of family brokers/go-betweens. First, the practitioner must remain aware that the family bilingual communicator will inadvertently or consciously be screening and possibly culturally modifying the communications. In Case 4.1, the López family daughter did not relay the venereal-disease–based aspect of her father's dementia diag-nosis. It took a subsequent visit by the clinic's bilingual/bicultural staff member to bridge the communication gap. Second, it is important not to place family members in conflict-of-interest positions. The family go-between, being the sole inter-cultural communicator on the scene, can be put in just such a spot. Third, the family go-between may not have sufficient technical background to transmit the key nuances included in the medical and scientific information related to the elder's specific diagnosis.

As indicated earlier, there is no intent to exclude the family's own bilingual/ bicultural communicator from the overall intercultural engagement process. On the contrary, these people can play an integral role in assisting to mobilize the family's own coping capabilities and understandings about dementing illness. These bilingual go-betweens can be invaluable assets to the overall intercultural communication process. For example, as they come to understand dementing illness, they can serve as internal family educators. However, this and other functions are best performed if the go-betweens are left in their usual family roles rather than made to play the part of adjunct practitioners. Moreover, professionals or providers and their parent organizations cannot excuse themselves from their responsibility to meet the intercultural communication challenge at the appropriate level of professionalism.

PRIMARY CAREGIVER, ROLES, FAMILY DECISION MAKING

It is sometimes difficult to immediately identify the primary caregiver within many ethnically diverse families. This is especially so where there is an extended family with many persons involved in the caretaking activity, possibly in many different homes, some nearby and some at a distance. The dementia-affected elder may even be rotated through these different households, each of which at some time has the major responsibility for the ADLs and IADLs. Sorting out all of the persons and the roles may take some time. There are some ethnocultural groups, such as the ethnic Chinese, for which the knowledgeable practitioner will be aware that the eldest son and his wife are expected to play this primary caregiver role, at least to the extent that major decisions have to be made. This is not always the case with other ethnic groups. For example among some Latinos, the spouse will ostensibly be identified with the caregiving role. However, if it is the male spouse, he may lack some of the skills required to provide ADL support to the dementia-affected elder. In such cases a daughter or a more distant female relative, or even a neighbor, may become the hands-on caregiver. The husband may make the overall decisions, but the bathing, toileting, and meal preparation—for all intents and purposes, the major portion of the primary care—may reside in these other persons.

There is a variety of caregiving arrangements to be found among ethnically diverse families, not all of which can be described here at length. As was noted in Chapter 5, the issue for the professional and provider is to be prepared to enter the ethnically diverse client family environment from a different cultural perspective. The key point that practitioners need to keep in mind is that, in working with ethnically diverse clients, they are most often entering a situation in which a collectivist type decision-making or decision-influencing process is at work. There will be many different care network members who will be influencing the individual who is finally identified as the primary caregiver. The caregiver in turn will engage these social network members in regard to key decisions that need to be made regarding the dementia-affected elder. This network could include friends and neighbors, or native healers or practitioners. Cases 5.3 and 5.4 in Chapter 5, along with Cases 6.1 and 6.2 in Chapter 6, could all serve as examples in which the caregivers sought assistance outside the family from indigenous sources.

As discussed in these earlier chapters, especially Chapter 5, the intercultural-focused practitioner has to be flexible and accept the extended decision network process. Certainly, the multiplicity of network people involved and the delays that often occur before a decision is reached or an action taken can seem to slow the overall careplanning process down. At the same time, the culturally attuned practitioner can make good use of the process to eventually bring a more stable care situation for the dementia-affected individual. As noted in Chapter 5, the professional or provider can take the perspective that many individuals can become integrally involved, once a solution is agreed on. For example, the many hands can be mobilized to provide respite on a rotating basis for the identified primary caregiver. Moreover, like it or not, the practitioner interacting with these larger social networks will need to assist some of the members in coming to grips with the realities regarding the dementia-affected person in their midst.

Employing the Cultural Mapping/Intercultural Assessment Checklist, Step 3, the practitioner documents the family/significant other network involved. Where indicated, the professional or provider can implement the eco-mapping component of the documentation of the relationships involved in the ethnically diverse social network that is encountered (see Chapter 5, Figure 5.1). Beginners might physically draw the eco map, whereas experienced practitioners might use the concept more automatically to determine the positives and negatives present in the situation they encounter. At the same time, experienced professionals and providers might consider the benefits of formally charting the client system progress relative to the cultural mapping process so that other practitioners entering the case situation will be able to refer to the documented information if necessary.

THE VALUES ARENA

As noted in Chapter 6, the target ethnic client group's values will remain in the more private sectors of the members' daily lives. Regardless, the professional or provider will find that many value indicators emerge within the already-discussed cultural mapping areas, Box 9.1, Step 3, the group's language and communicational processes, Step 4, the ethnic group's intrafamily and significant other relationships, Step 5. The practitioner must immediately begin to note whatever can be learned relative to the client group's beliefs, customary expectations, and normative outlooks, as these outlooks express themselves within the intercultural engagement process.

As also noted earlier, the task is especially crucial with regard to identifying the ethnic group members' understanding of dementing illness, particularly to highlight where these understandings may rest along the acculturation continuum. For example, the ethnically diverse caregivers at the more traditional end of the spectrum might begin to talk about the possibility that the source of the dementing behaviors is an outside force or that the dementia can be cured through spiritual or natural healing, such as in Cases 5.2, 5.3, 6.1, and 6.2. Those with a more acculturated outlook might immediately absorb the medical and scientific content being provided by the practitioner. At the same time, the professional or provider must be ready to document a mixed acculturation profile, such as in Case 6.1, in which Mrs. Ortega, the caregiver, understood the medical and scientific explanation of her husband's Alzheimer's condition but nonetheless sought solace from traditional practices, as did the family members in Case 6.2, the Landis family. The identification of the ethnic group members' perceptions and expectations in regard to culturally acceptable help-seeking and help-accepting attitudes and behaviors can be made in a similar fashion.

The task is at once interesting and formidable. The determination of value perspectives is interesting because it challenges the practitioner to know the culture backward and forward. It also challenges the practitioner to recognize how culture is modified over time. Finally, it is challenging because it requires the professional or provider to bypass stereotypes and accurately place the target ethnic group members at the correct point on the acculturation continuum with regard to their value outlooks and normative expectations in a number of different social environments: at home, in the workplace, in the clinic or agency setting, or elsewhere. Values, beliefs, and normative expectations may get "played out" differently in each setting. The professional or provider must be able to handle the possibly different underlying responses by the ethnic group members relative to where along the acculturation process the clients may be at the moment. This task is formidable for the same reasons. Considerable effort is required to appropriately identify the cultural variations that are seen while at the same time avoiding falling into stereotypes regarding any one ethnic group or individual within the group.

At times the professional or provider, especially the beginner, will find the values documentation arena somewhat elusive. The ethnic group members' attitudinal and normative perspectives will most likely not be overtly declared. Therefore, the practitioner will be dependent on behaviors or statements that may reflect underlying views. As has been noted, the task will ease as relationship between the practitioner and the ethnically diverse client deepens. The rapport and trust-building processes outlined in Chapters 4 and 7 will greatly facilitate the professional's or provider's entry into the ethnic group members' values domain. Always, though, the recommendation remains that practitioners develop a written or internalized structured format that permits them to review and sift what is heard and observed for its meaning relative to the group members' underlying worldviews. Without such a framework, the information could emerge as a jumble of ideas drawn from tradition, from the host society, and from the ethnic client group's own interpretations—all present simultaneously, but seemingly without order.

Order, however, is present. People from ethnically diverse groups in the United States, just as other segments of the population identified as coming from the mainstream, act on the basis of deeply held convictions when it comes to coping with the crises stemming from dementing illness. The coping may appear inadequate or even dysfunctional to the outsider, but the close observer will begin to find patterns, and it is these value-based patterns that the interculturally oriented professional or provider needs to identify and document.

There is an additional aspect of the values arena that must be addressed. There are times when the ethnically diverse client group members may find themselves in conflict. They will see themselves as caught between their own culture-of-origin value sets and those of the host society as reflected by the professional and dementia-care service values. This can lead to what was noted in Chapters 4 and 7 as *cultural paralysis,* in which the caregiver, torn by different mandates, appears immobilized. The situation is generally delicate but often workable. The professional or provider must, however, demonstrate patience and understanding while attempting to move the situation ahead.

The deadlock between value systems is broken through a variety of practical steps. For example, as indicated in Chapter 5, the practitioner can bargain with the ethnically diverse client, providing the opportunity for the primary caregiver or the family members to try out their traditional ways while at the same time asking them to take one or several steps toward the orthodox system of services. In this approach, both the ethnically diverse client's and the practitioner's concerns for the dementia-affected patient receive recognition. The intercultural engagement process usually takes hold when the target client group members see that the professional or provider has a direct interest in the well-being of their family members. This interest does not take the form of altruistic statements or the reiteration of the dementia-care organization's mission; rather, it is expressed through concrete actions that indicate the actual merging of different value systems to meet immediate needs of the dementia-affected elder and the caregiving family members. Once again, all of these actions on the part of professionals or providers does not mean that they are to give up communicating their basic scientific understandings of dementing illness. Instead, the approach is to transculturate the practitioner's outlooks to blend them into the framework of the ethnic client group coming for service. The concept of transculturation refers to the process of going beyond simple translation from English to a designated ethnic group language. Through the process of transculturation the practitioner ensures that the content being communicated has the following features (Butcher, 1982; Helms, 1992; Lonner, 1981). First, the information being communicated describes something that has behavioral correlates within the target ethnic group members' experience. In context of the discussion in this text, this implies that the signs and symptoms of a dementing condition would be recognized by the ethnically diverse clients. Second, the signs and symptoms would be organized into a conceptual framework that could be understood by the ethnic group client group members. Third, the actual terms used to explain the signs and symptoms of dementing illness would be drawn from the colloquial or more commonly used language of the ethnic group members. The notion of transculturation is elaborated in Chapter 12.

THE ISSUE OF CULTURAL ASSESSMENT DISTORTING FACTORS

Inextricably bound with cultural elements are the social status factors discussed in full in Chapter 6. The social status elements that influence ethnically diverse populations are fallouts from lack of access to appropriate dementia-care resources, conditions of prejudice and discrimination, and the fact that modern-day immigrants to the United States have entered a highly technological society that prizes formal education in English. All of these factors in some manner have left some impact on ethnically diverse populations. Ethnically diverse individuals and their fellow family members have likewise experienced the impact of these forces at very personal levels.

However, the effects of these different social status-related elements are not uniform. Generalizations are hard to draw without knowing the individual situation. Therefore, the professional or practitioner engaged in the cultural mapping process must determine, what, if any, of the factors listed in Step 6 of the Cultural Mapping/ Intercultural Assessment Checklist have an impact on the ethnically diverse family client group being targeted for services. To be effective, this determination must be drawn separately and not mixed into the cultural components assessment.

Lower socioeconomic status may be the major determinant for a specific ethnically diverse family's eligibility for services rather than their cultural attitudes and, as indicated in the Harris case (Case 7.2), the residual effects of prejudice, expressed as racism, can influence the current limited world of the dementia-affected ethnically diverse elder. The situation in the Harris case was not one of ethnic orientation. Similarly, lower literacy rather than resistance to learning about dementing illness, can likewise play a role in the manner in which dementia focused communications will be understood. Case 7.4 provides some illustrative content related to the influence of schooling. By making the appropriate distinctions, the practitioner refines the cultural map being drawn, sorting the information into the appropriate compartments belonging to cultural or society status factors.

REINFORCING CULTURAL MAPPING THROUGH PROBLEM SOLVING

Because there are many different types of problems found among dementia-affected ethnically diverse populations, a structured problem-solving strategy must be incorporated within the proposed intercultural engagement/cultural mapping approach suggested. The strategy provides the opportunity for the professional or provider to implement a culturally relevant intervention while at the same time inculcating problem-solving skills within the target ethnic group. It also provides for reinforced learning at the ethnic client's cultural pace, and it enables the ethnic client to carry on after the culturally sensitive professional or provider might no longer be available. The approach likewise enables the practitioner to gain the sufficient process and client engagement time through which to implement the various steps or phases of cultural mapping within the specific situation being encountered. As used here, the intervention strategy is a modification of Berlin and Fowkes's (1983) formulation for client intervention, given the acronym *LEARN*. In its present application, the LEARN approach includes the following operational principles.

First, the professional or provider *locates* the client group within the target ethnic group members' own culture. Here the practitioner makes the appropriate cultural history assessments and identifies the language(s) of reference to be used, the traditional interactional format to be found, the customs to be followed, and values held. The practitioner also identifies and *localizes* the key care problems facing the dementia-affected elder and the elder's family/significant other informal network. As indicated at various points in this discussion, the expectation is that the practitioner must be both culturally competent and dementia capable

Second, at a pace suitable to the inclusion of both the cultural features of the situation and the pressing needs arising from the dementing illness condition, the professional or provider *engages* the caregiver and\or family member/significant others in both problem-solving approaches relative to the service systems being found within one's service region and in blending the new approaches to their own traditional outlooks. Here the practitioner actively *educates* the target ethnic group clients so that the family members/significant others can gain problem-solving success under guidance and direction.

Third, the practitioner assists the caregiver and family network/significant other group to *assess* and *appraise* their newly gained problem-solving learning. Wherever the opportunity lends itself, links to the family's own cultural attitudes and beliefs, along with the ethnic care network's customs and practices, are not just permitted but actively incorporated into the appraisals and assessments made.

Fourth, the practitioner enables the caregiver and family members to *repeat* their success, *reinforcing* and *reintegrating* the focused problem-solving learning acquired along with those aspects supportive of both the elder's and the ethnic care network members' traditional, bicultural, and acculturated orientations. The reinforcement is a major contributor to long-term problem-solving learning, especially in the arena of dementing illness, where the problems may not only persist but also increase in intensity over a period of years.

Finally, the practitioner enables the caregiver and family/significant others involved in the care of the dementia-affected elder to *normalize* their more newly acquired problem-solving capabilities. The LEARN approach enables the target ethnic client group members to overlay their culturally compatible help-seeking and help-accepting dementia care strategies with those obtained through contact with the practitioner.

The strategy of establishing a mutual assistance/monitoring schedule between the professional or provider and the target ethnic client group is a key tool for the reinforcing of a successful intercultural relationship. However, as understated as the above outline may appear, there are some important considerations to take into account. At the beginning stages of establishing contact with the family, it is extremely important to teach and train the family in such a way as to establish a mutually workable arrangement. As has been noted earlier, rushing into the formal side of dementia-care information without working through the cultural subtleties present in the target ethnic group situation can be a prescription for failure.

The combined aspect of merging a problem-solving strategy with cultural mapping brings with it some acknowledged stressors. The fact of the matter is that at any given moment the professional or provider will more than likely be involved in the management of multiple cases, with all at different stages of the dementing illness process. Some families will be in crisis, others will have medical emergencies, others will have had an onset of a new behavior manifestation. Moreover, the practitioner seeking to extend the culturally relevant strategy to the existing services may find a "patchwork" type of formal service systems response. What can be added to these elements of the situation is the present scarcity of interculturally trained and knowledgeable professional providers working in the field of dementia.

At the same time, the problem-solving intervention approach woven into the overall cultural mapping strategy allows the professional or provider to cut through some of the difficulties to be encountered and to tailor the intervention to the specific needs and learning abilities of the caregiver and/or the family members/significant others caring for the dementia-affected patient. In some instances the intervention calls primarily for information and referral to a specific array of services, such as day care and respite assistance. In other cases, depending on the situational requirement, the practitioner will need to actually model the activity for the ethnically diverse client. In any of the cases, the joint problem solving–cultural mapping approach provides for intercultural relevancy. Box 9.2 highlights the key components of the LEARN strategy.

CONSISTENCY OF EFFORT: A FURTHER ASSET

Whatever the specific form the intercultural engagement method takes, it must be established at the onset of ethnic family contact and be followed through consistently.

STEP 1. The practitioner *locates* the ethnically diverse group members within cultural identifications. Key dementia care problems are *linked* to resources within the social environment encompassable to them.

STEP 2. The practitioner *engages* the ethnically diverse client group in a problem-solving strategy blending traditional cultural and host society resources. This strategy is tested out *experientially* by the ethnic client group members.

STEP 3. The practitioner assists the ethnic client group members to *assess* and *appraise* their performance.

STEP 4. The practitioner provides *reinforcements* for the problem solving gains made. Where possible the successes are *repeated,* providing additional reinforcement and *reintegration* of the learning experiences.

STEP 5. The practitioner enables the ethnically diverse caregiver and significant others to *normalize* their newly acquired problem solving capabilities.

Box 9.2 *LEARN* intercultural problem solving formulation.

This consistency over time provides for a more successful practice. There are many techniques that can be used to reinforce continuity of contact. For example, the professional or provider can make a point of remembering the dementia-affected elder's or the caregiver's birthdays. To convey continuing interest, the practitioner can also make a point to be aware of culturally specific celebrations or religious holidays and observances. Should a staff change take place, the professional or provider who had established the relationship with the ethnically diverse clients should make every effort to personally broker the incoming practitioner into the relationship. This can be accomplished through an in-person contact; by phone; or by a written message, perhaps enclosed in a personalized card. All of these actions communicate a continuity of interest to the ethnically diverse family being served. In essence, the outgoing interculturally competent practitioner acts in a cultural broker mode. Continuity is also reinforced through the ongoing monitoring not only of the service plan but also of the intercultural communication breakdowns. An underlying premise of intercultural contact is that one relates on a more basic and feeling–sharing level rather than simply carrying out a professional task or assignment.

STEPS TO ENSURE CROSS-CULTURAL ENGAGEMENT

There are a number of ways in which the professional or provider can ensure the maintenance of cross-cultural competency within the ethnically diverse client–practitioner engagement process.

1. **The practitioner must be prepared to apply, and actually reapply, the acculturation continuum as an integral part of the intervention process.** As outlined in Chapter 2, culture is subject to changes over time and process.

Therefore, the professional or practitioner must be prepared to alter some of the cultural assessments made as new information emerges, as new people enter the careplan arrangements, or as the target ethnic group clients themselves change and gain new insights. The formulation allows for flexibility and in fact encourages the ongoing development of additional insights within the intercultural engagement process.

2. **The practitioner must be prepared to undertake a comprehensive, rather than a cursory or partial, cultural assessment.** Admittedly, there are often time constraints that must be considered. Certainly, if the ethnically diverse client and the professional or provider come together at the point of a crisis, the crisis has to be dealt with first, particularly to meet the needs of the dementia-affected person. However, on resolving the immediate concerns, the practitioner must return to the cultural assessment task. As was noted throughout Chapter 3, the gathering of information to complete the cultural assessment cannot be left to be completed after all other work has been done.

3. **The practitioner must be ready for the fact that, in reality, the cultural information from the ethnically diverse client group members and their situation will arrive in a "scrambled" form.** As indicated above, people live their culture rather than conceptualize it. Therefore, to make the cultural mapping process work easily, it is incumbent on the professional or provider to organize the information as it is provided. In this respect, the cultural assessment process is no different from any other assessment undertaken by the practitioner. He or she must have the capability to organize information, however it is provided, into meaningful components and then extend to a coherent treatment plan to the client. The difference in the cultural assessment lies in the kind of content that serves as basis for the assessment and careplan.

4. **The LEARN strategy suggested above may resemble the problem-solving models used in a variety of disciplines and provider settings. Its uniqueness lies in both the cultural content areas that are emphasized and in the client education, empowerment, and modeling functions that are built into the approach.** The LEARN approach assumes that many ethnically diverse client group members will (a) be unfamiliar with the culture of dementia care systems and services and (b) if somewhat knowledgeable about services, will nonetheless be unfamiliar with the intricate cultural nuances of how to actually access and subsequently navigate the systems successfully. In this context, therefore, the professional or provider has to be prepared to "teach" systems-appraisal skills, reinforcing and reintegrating the knowledge and experience gained. The cultural alienness of formal dementia care provider systems cannot be understated, and, in many instances, it is this cultural alienness, rather than a lack of intelligence, initiative, or motivation on the part of the ethnically diverse client, that is the barrier to accessing services or following through with aspects of the careplan.

END NOTE

The true power of the cultural assessment is realized when it is linked to all the other information available about the dementia-affected elder's condition and the overall caregiving situation. The cultural mapping approach avoids sending inappropriate or sure-to-be-misunderstood diagnostic and/or careplan messages to the caregivers and the significant others engaged with the dementia-affected elder. Unfortunately, because of the lack of awareness throughout the dementia-care field about the significant role that culture plays in the family members' and significant others' responses to dementing illness, cultural assessment tends to be relegated to an afterthought. The suggestion here is to put cultural assessment at the forefront. The cultural mapping principles discussed above provide a ready tool for the professional or provider. They can be applied to any evaluative situation. Cultural mapping can also be made applicable all ethnic groups.

Part Three

Supporting Intercultural Competency Development

The adult social day center activities volunteer was talking to a fellow volunteer from another program.

> Case A. "It finally happened. I don't remember quite when it did, but the clientele of our center are different now than they were a few years ago."
>
> "What do you mean, 'different'?"
>
> "Well, we've put different kinds of foods on the menu. We've hired staff who can work with our clients from different cultures. We have a Spanish-speaking nurse and a bilingual Chinese community outreach worker. I guess that the effort paid off. I wasn't always sure. For a long time I didn't think it would. We kept trying and trying, but nobody seemed to come. All those meetings I used to go to and still no Hispanic or Chinese families would come—for the longest time."

For the activities volunteer, everything finally seemed to be coming together at the day care center. Ethnic diversity was being accomodated by the program. However, the ethnoculturally diverse clientele did not just happen to come into the day center program by chance. Had the center's director been speaking instead, the comments would have been quite different. The director had taken a number of steps to bring the day care center to its present culture-friendly (Aranda, 1990) level of intercultural engagement to include two ethnically diverse groups in addition to the mainstream English-speaking clientele (Goodman, 1989). The organization's manager had taken leadership in producing what Fine (1995, p. 40) calls a *multiculturally transforming supportive environment.* Considerable planning and community liaison activity had laid the groundwork for the present interculturally attuned state of the organization. In addition, the director had worked intensively with the board of directors to bring budget and resource support to the cross-cultural outreach effort. The center's administrative and direct-service personnel, each within their individual areas of responsibility, had also collaborated to reach the present level of development of the center's multicultural capability.

Part Three focuses on the broader aspects of practitioner and/or parent organization preparedness that not only serve to embellish the cultural mapping/intercultural engagement process but also help make it an integral part of the organization's everyday operations. A working premise throughout Part Three is that intercultural engagement in dementia service cannot be left solely as the responsibility of the individual professional or provider. The organization must actively participate in the process and do so at all of its different structural levels. Part Three brings the discussion around to the more macro or community-focused aspects of the cultural mapping/intercultural engagement strategy.

Chapter 10 highlights how the organization can examine itself from top to bottom to incorporate the elements necessary to its own structure and process that will enable it to enter the intercultural engagement effort from a position of internal strength. Throughout the discussion, the organization's competency with respect to dementing illness evaluation and intervention are assumed. The focus is rather on the key *cultural attunement* factors that will enable the organization to demonstrate its intercultural engagement competency and to interact with its multicultural environment. The chapter stresses the organizational elements that will enable the direct-care practitioner to focus on the needs of specifically targeted ethnocultural group clients.

Chapter 11 presents an overview of how both the organization as a whole, and the practitioner in particular, can link to and make use of the *cultural brokers* relative to the ethnocultural group being targeted for dementia-care services. As discussed in the chapter, the cultural-broker role complements both the organization's and the individual practitioner's intercultural engagement/cultural mapping activity with ethnically diverse populations. Basically, cultural brokers are people from the ethnic group itself as well as bilingual/bicultural individuals who serve as gatekeepers/links to the specific ethnic communities. It is often from this pool that the practitioner or the organization locates persons previously identified as the "ethnically diverse" members of the bicultural-pair. Techniques relevant to establishing longer term ties to cultural brokers are also discussed in this chapter. In examining the presence of cultural brokers it is important to recognize that the cultural brokers are not simply waiting there to be contacted. Rather, the professional and provider must gain an understanding of the skills needed to both cultivate and maintain the organizational and/or practitioner–cultural broker working relationship over time.

Chapter 12 explores still another vital aspect of the overall cultural mapping/intercultural engagement process undertaken by both the organization as a whole and the individual practitioner. This involves the development of culturally and linguistically appropriate informational materials and content for dissemination to ethnically diverse populations. The chapter discusses the techniques of both preparing and presenting dementia-focused content in the format preferred by the target ethnic group members.

Chapter 13 summarizes a number of both culturally directed outreach and networking strategies that are readily available to the dementia-care organization and the individual practitioner alike. Outreach activity takes a different form when it engages the organizational and agency infrastructure of the target ethnocultural community than when it targets ethnically diverse families for service recruitment purposes. The latter activity formed the core of the discussion for Parts One and Two. In Part Three the concept of outreach looks to interorganizational and practitioner peer relationship formation. However, the chapter assumes that for effective intercultural outreach to take place, the practitioner and the organization must have a solid grasp of the principles of cultural mapping outlined in Part One and summarized in Part Two.

As delineated in the chapter, intercultural networking is seen as a natural extension of outreach. This aspect of the ethnic community engagement process requires role consistency on the part of the professional or provider, as well as the continued support of the parent dementia-care organization. The differences between networking, outreach, and marketing activities are outlined.

Chapter 14 provides an overall summary of issues relative to the cultural mapping process. It also covers a number of issues beyond the capability of the present text to cover in any detail, but which nonetheless require attention if the process of intercultural engagement is to gain full institutional status within the field of dementia care. Perhaps dementia-care organizations and their shareholders, along with their managers, can come to see that new service populations are actually assets to their overall growth. Ethnically diverse groups are new dementia-care service markets that can enhance the organizational place within the overall region served. Part Three offers suggestions on how to move in this direction.

Chapter 10

The Interculturally Capable Agency: The Ideal

To adequately meet the needs of dementia-affected ethnically diverse populations, dementia-care organizations need to institutionalize cross-cultural capabilities within themselves (Applewhite, Wong, & Daly, 1991; Meyerson, 1994; Valle et al., 1989), that is, intercultural knowledge and skills must be made an everyday part of the life of the organization (Gentile, 1994; Thiederman, 1991). The reality, at this writing, is that much of the intercultural engagement activity with ethnically diverse populations is being carried out at the level of direct contact by professionals and providers. Here and there, organizations have geared themselves up to engage in the provision of cross-cultural dementia care, but the efforts are as yet scattered, varying from region to region. The premise of this portion of the discussion is that direct service staff who are carrying the intercultural engagement burden must have organizationwide support. To provide such support, the organization must (a) assess its preparedness for intercultural practice, (b) align its personnel for cross-cultural engagement, (c) redirect its mission and objectives, (d) allocate its resources to appropriately support the intercultural effort, (e) maintain its commitment to a steady presence in the target ethnic community, and (f) develop and deploy a self-monitoring processes to determine if it remains on track throughout the intercultural engagement process.

ORGANIZATIONAL PREPAREDNESS
FOR CULTURAL PRACTICE

It is one thing for the individual professional or provider to get the caregiver, the patient, and the family/significant other as a group ready to engage services. But if the ethnically diverse clients arrive at the practitioner's organizational setting and the necessary cultural sensitivity is not present among the different components of the organization, setbacks can occur, and the overall careplan can be undermined.

> Case 10.1a. The bilingual Vietnamese American social worker at the Alzheimer's clinic had been working with the Nguyen family for some time. First, the practitioner helped the family members to see that the elder Mrs. Nguyen seemed to have the symptoms of a dementing illness. Second, the staff member had won family acceptance for a full diagnostic evaluation for dementia at the clinic. The elder Mr. Nguyen, as his children said, was from the old ways. He had never heard of Alzheimer's disease and felt his wife was better off with the help the family could give. The children indicated that he was really ashamed to have to get help outside the family. "This was not proper," he said. As Mrs. Nguyen's condition worsened, he finally agreed to go to the clinic appointment.

In setting up the clinic appointment, the Vietnamese American social worker had made many advance arrangements for the Nguyens' reception at the clinic. Because the practitioner was the only bilingual staff member, part of the arrangement was that she would have double duty translating throughout the process.

The Nguyen family arrived at the appointed time. Unfortunately, a major traffic delay caused the social worker to be late. She was able to call ahead and speak with the elder Mr. Nguyen on her cellular phone, assuring him that she would come to the clinic as soon as the traffic cleared. When she arrived an hour later, the Nguyen family had left, and the diagnostic evaluation process had been cut short.

Needless to say the bilingual/bicultural social worker was quite upset by the outcome and determined to understand what had happened. With careful work she put a number of the important pieces of the story together.

> Case 10.1b. Mr. Nguyen, his wife (the patient), and the adult children had come on time for the appointment. Because of the Vietnamese social worker's absence, another social work staff member was assigned the intake interview responsibilities. As he was not bilingual Vietnamese speaking, he engaged the eldest son and asked him to help out in the interview. The process had gone on for a few minutes, and the social worker noted that the son, instead of answering the items, kept deferring to the elder Mr. Nguyen, even in regard to confirmation of basic demographic information that had been secured by the Vietnamese-American social worker in advance. In the middle of the session he noticed that Mr. Nguyen became quite flustered as the son began verifying Mrs. Nguyen's symptoms and behaviors, which included incontinence and some combativeness. At this point, Mr. Nguyen stood up and indicated that the family had to leave, which they did.

Although it is not always easy for the agency to prepare itself for an ethnically diverse clientele, some organizational preplanning for the new ethnically diverse clientele is in order. In the case of the Nguyen family, the Alzheimer's clinic had only one Vietnamese American social worker. When events beyond her control interfered with her presence, a less interculturally prepared substitute intake worker moved into the situation. Although not bicultural Vietnamese himself, he did observe some of the family dynamics, including both the bilingual son's and Mr. Nguyen's discomfort. However, he did not know what to make of it. Mr. Nguyen's action precluded any effort to find out in the session itself.

In reconstructing what had occurred, the bilingual/bicultural Vietnamese practitioner first went back to the family and confirmed what she had suspected. Mr. Nguyen had already been on edge about going to the appointment, and when he had to reveal what he considered personal family matters to a stranger he confirmed his views that this was not appropriate and decided that they all had to leave. She recognized that Mr. Nguyen was perhaps a personal extreme example of some deeply held Vietnamese cultural values. Her own father still held similar outlooks but not to the same extent.

To follow up the situation, the Vietnamese practitioner asked that the agency's practice of reconfirming demographic and patient symptom information be changed. She made further arrangements for the health history and preliminary health examination to be conducted in the home. For this she took with her the clinic's nurse practitioner, who administered the noninvasive procedures, measuring Mrs. Nguyen's blood pressure, and so on. But when it came to the Alzheimer's clinic itself, beyond suggesting that some training be instituted to familiarize the staff with the Vietnamese culture, the practitioner was not sure what to do.

Cultural Practice Preparedness: A Further Look

More could be said about the individual aspects of the Nguyen family cases. However, it is more important at this juncture to take a look at its organizational implications. First, the Alzheimer's clinic is to be complimented for having hired an able bilingual/ bicultural Vietnamese American practitioner, who seemed to have made inroads into the Vietnamese community. However, a systems assessment reveals that too much of the intercultural engagement effort appeared to rely on her. There were some notable gaps in the overall staff-level readiness and awareness of different aspects of the Vietnamese culture. In line with the Vietnamese practitioner's observation, some form of staffwide intercultural engagement training seemed to be in order (Brislin & Yoshida, 1994; Cushner & Brislin, 1996; Harris & Moran, 1987). For example, even the simple delaying of the clinic intake session and offering the Nguyen family refreshments until the Vietnamese social worker could arrive might have helped. In any event, a broad conceptual base about Vietnamese culture had to be created within clinic staff, along with practical suggestions about what to do in difficult situations (Brownlee, 1978).

Second, the role of administration in the overall process was not clear. Certainly the clinic's managers had much to with the hiring of the bilingual/bicultural social worker. At the same time there is much more that the clinic managers could have done to get ready for the eventual influx of ethnically diverse clients. Existing protocols could have been modified to make them more culturally friendly and flexible (Brownlee, 1978; pp. 248–252). For example, permission could have been given to do as much of the evaluative work as possible in the field.

Third, a role could be inferred for the clinic's governing board (Alzheimer's Disease and Related Disorders Association, 1994; Valle, 1989). In this case a series of questions would need to be asked. How much investment was the governing board making in supporting the budding service effort to the Vietnamese community? In what way was the board itself linked to this ethnic group at its own level of operation? For example, had offers been extended to include as board members prominent members of the Vietnamese community as well as caregivers? Continuing in the same vein, how was the governing board upgrading its own understandings about engaging the organization in intercultural work? Was there some form of intercultural training taking place at the board level?

Somewhere along the line the dementia-care organization as a whole has to enter into proposed intercultural engagement activity. Ideally, to support the intercultural dementia-care work, a number of components must be brought together in an organizationwide capabilities development effort (Alzheimer's Disease and Related Disorders Association, 1994; Valle, 1989). These elements include the following.

1. Incorporation of interculturally proficient personnel at all levels of the organization. This step also encompasses the ongoing availability of training efforts and staff development programs to upgrade the intercultural knowledge and skills of the present complement of staff.
2. Redirection of the organizational mission, working objectives, and policies.
3. Reallocation of budget and other resources to support the intercultural effort.
4. Maintenance of a steady presence in the community, including the opening of new ethnically diverse markets and the transfer of dementia-capable technology to the target ethnic community.
5. Establishment of self-monitoring and other evaluative mechanisms to maintain the overall effort on target.

INTERCULTURAL ALIGNMENT OF ORGANIZATIONAL PERSONNEL

Dementia-care organizations, whether large or small, whether service-directed or research-focused, or program-planning and service supportive in nature, are generally complex. Similar to other organizations, they have a number of subcomponents that are designed to establish their overall viability in their work environments as well as their continuance over time. For example, dementia-care organizations tend to have several staffing levels, including some form of governing board, managers, and the line staff that directly engage client populations. In proprietary organizations the governing board may be the owners. The issue is that most organizations have a group of people who oversee the organization's direction, another group that administers its ongoing functions, and still another group charged with the day-to-day hands-on operations.

Each of these personnel groupings is in itself much more elaborate than will be portrayed in this discussion. For example, administration may contain many different hierarchical levels and subdivisions. One can find the executive officer, assistant to the executive, department or unit heads, and so forth. Line staff may likewise include considerable personnel variation with regard to the different disciplines represented: medicine, psychology, social work, nursing, and a host of allied health professions. The line staff level may also have its own hierarchy; for example, there may be the professionals, the support staff, the aides, and so on. These complexities are present regardless of the size and scope of dementia-care organizations. However, that is not the point of the discussion. The purpose here remains how to best infuse cross-ethnic capabilities throughout the total organization, regardless of how it is structured, and thereby be ready to serve ethnically diverse clienteles (Aranda, 1990; Cunningham, 1991–1992; Fine, 1995; Green & Monohan, 1984; Ham, 1987; Holmes et al., 1979; R. J. Taylor, Neighbors, & Broman, 1989; Valle, 1989, 1992a, 1992b).

Multicultural or Culture-Specific Capabilities

The question of whether the organization should be multicultural or culture-specific in scope was addressed earlier in the discussion. The answer is that the organization must develop both sets of competencies (Harris & Moran, 1987; also see the introduction to Part One of this book). Most service environments or regions where dementia-care organizations operate are multicultural. As indicated earlier, dementing illness in some form affects cultural populations across the spectrum of their diversity, although it may affect each ethnic group in a differential manner. Therefore, the likelihood is present that linguistically and culturally diverse people will be requiring some form of services. The organization has to be ready to respond to this diversity.

At the same time, the everyday realities of service provision dictate the targeting of specific ethnic groups for services. Most often, there is a scarcity of interculturally oriented and trained staff. Moreover, those staff who are so trained will be primarily bilingual/bicultural with respect to the targeted ethnocultural groups. Occasionally there will be trilingual personnel, for example, Chinese American staff who may speak English and the two main Chinese dialects, Mandarin and Cantonese. On rare occasions there may even be multilingual staff. However, individuals with these skills will be quite rare. The shortage of personnel resources, as well as other organizational factors, leads organizations to target specific ethnic groups for intercultural dementia-care engagement. Each organization, therefore, must resolve its own priorities with regard to its multicultural environment and the manner in which specific ethnic groups requesting or needing services are addressed. It is not that personnel cannot learn new cultural ways, but rather that they have to match the means and context of the target ethnic populations (Banks, 1995).

Regardless of the scope of the organizational response, whether more multicultural or more ethnic specific, the organization is still left with the need to infuse intercultural engagement/cultural mapping capabilities at each of its different personnel levels. Without such an orientation, the organization will continue to use only its present mainstream culturally oriented assessment and intervention approaches. These strategies may be workable for the mainstream English-speaking clientele; however, they may be unsuitable for clients with other linguistic and cultural backgrounds.

GOVERNING BOARD

In a manner of speaking, the governing boards of dementia-care organizations are often diversified, although not ethnically. The boards are diversified in the context of the mixes of individual skills and backgrounds that were brought in to enhance the organization's fiscal strength, its credibility within the mainstream society, and so on. In the dementia-care arena one often finds governing boards composed of contributors, people with specialized professional backgrounds, such as business executives, medical, legal, and financial experts and, in the case of community-based dementia-care organizations, one also finds caregivers of dementia-affected individuals often serving on the board. The governing boards generally know well how to identify, recruit, and involve likely candidates whose presence, participation, and contributions will directly benefit the organization in terms of its stature and fiscal soundness. From an intercultural capability development perspective, the board member recruitment and retention skills can be extended to include ethnically diverse candidates. However, for this to happen throughout the dementia-care field two substantive steps must take place. First, the governing boards must make their own internal ethnic diversity a priority. Second, they must actively redirect their recruitment and retention strategies to involve ethnically diverse colleagues from within their working environment (*Multicultural Outreach Program Manual*, 1994, Sec. 6, pp. 1–4).

Admittedly, the second step will take considerable time and effort, especially if the search is starting out at the ground floor and if the board lacks familiarity with the ethnic group(s) being targeted for inclusion. However, the board can often turn to its line-level practitioner staff, who may already be engaged with ethnically diverse clientele. These staff members will both know the community and be able to suggest potential candidates. Linkages with the cultural brokers, as discussed in Chapter 11, will provide the governing board additional avenues through which to access specific ethnic groups. Other governing boards that have been successful in attaining ethnic diversification also can be solicited for guidance.

Proprietary governing boards and some publicly funded local, state, or federal organizations present a special problem. There may not be a governing board as generally constituted within the not-for-profit dementia-care organization sector. In the case of the proprietary organization, the governing board could be the owner of the shareholders. For the public organization, the governing board could be the legislature or an appointed or elected executive. However structured, none of these organizations is prohibited from forming intercultural advisory panels. These intercultural advisory panels could take on roles similar to not-for-profit governing boards around the cultural engagement issues. With some modifications in technique and purpose, ethnically diverse governing-board–type input can be made a regular component of the proprietary or public sector dementia-care organizations.

Organization's Managers

The organization's managerial level presents a different type of intercultural challenge. Here the diversity must be incorporated in the same manner that administrative personnel are usually hired and moved into positions within the organization.

However, the current organizational managers need to revise the approaches they already know with regard to the recruitment and retention of administrators and apply them, giving priority to securing interculturally competent personnel. Obviously, intercultural competence priorities have to be set early on in the process and recruitment strategies likewise put into place. There are organizations both within and outside of dementia care that have found interculturally competent management-level personnel. If nowhere else, the marketing and advertising industry is taking steps to target and reach ethnically and linguistically diverse groups. These organizations can be collectively tapped for their intercultural expertise.

There is an added benefit when the organizational management reflects the service area's diversity. The ethnoculturally diverse client group is more apt to engage an organization that is so structured (Green & Monohan, 1984; Harris & Moran, 1987; Valle, 1989). In other words, the client group that sees images of itself at different levels of the organizational structure is more culturally attracted to use the organization's services. This is not to say that having bilingually and biculturally capable administrators will automatically resolve all of the problems relative to engaging ethnically diverse clients in the dementia-care arena; the issues are not so simplistically resolved. Rather, the presence of ethnically diverse competence at the management level of the organization provides additional support to the direct-service line staff. In this context the direct-contact staff know they do not have to carry the total intercultural contact burden. The presence of intercultural management competence also serves as a resource for the governing board in its own search for diversity. After all, the board's interaction with organizational staff is usually at the top managerial levels, and it is these organizational administrators who can move the intercultural agenda forward (Harris & Moran, 1987, pp. 100–120).

Direct-Service Staff

The line staff present still another intercultural challenge for the organization. As noted, this may be where the major proportion of the organization's intercultural competence resides. It is important, therefore, not to overburden the interculturally capable staff members already at work in the ethnocultural arena. However, because these staff members often have information that is valuable to the total organization, there are some approaches that can be used to make optimum use of their capabilities (Harris & Moran, 1987, pp. 164–165). For example, some of the present responsibilities of the interculturally capable staff could lightened, and part of the staff members' time could be reassigned to providing their expertise to the other sectors of the dementia-care organization. Another strategy that is always available is to search for and hire additional cross-culturally capable practitioners to further enhance the organization's ethnically diverse dementia-care service.

Personnel Training and Development at All Levels

Internal training efforts to upgrade staff and board members' knowledge and skills on many topics related to dementing illness are commonplace. Cross-cultural capability building could likewise be incorporated into the different facets of the organization (Brislin & Yoshida, 1994; Cushner & Brislin, 1996; Pang & Barba, 1995; Pang, Gay, & Stanley, 1995). This intercultural training can take the form of organizational retreats, workshops, periodic educational sessions, and consultations, along with the provision for staff and board members to attend external meetings and conferences. Structured supervision conducted within the organization, apart from the supervision directed to administrative oversight, could also be put to the intercultural skills-upgrading purpose. Again, use can also be made of the cultural brokers discussed in Chapter 11 to assist with cultural training. Additionally, there are written, audio, and visual media products that could be used in the organization's internal training efforts. From an overall perspective, the organization's directors can take several steps to put their intercultural training and staff development house in order. First, the dementia-care organization's directors can make an inventory of the organization's present intercultural capabilities relative to all of its operational levels—the governing board, administration, and direct-service staff—to determine what needs to be done. Second, the directors can devise an immediate and long-range intercultural training plan for the organization as a whole and its different components. Third, the directors can implement the intercultural engagement plan. It is recognized that in implementing their intercultural staff-and-board-development effort, organizations will most likely mix and match different approaches to maximize the resources available to them. The important point is that dementia-care organizations put into place the kind of intercultural staff development programs to extend services to greater numbers of linguistically and culturally diverse populations.

REDIRECTION OF ORGANIZATIONAL MISSION AND OBJECTIVES

Implicit in the development of intercultural capabilities among the different sectors of the organization's personnel is the restructuring of the mission and operational objectives (*Multicultural Outreach Program Manual,* 1994, Sec. 6.3, 7.3). As administrators and board members know, redirecting the organization's mission and objectives appears deceptively simple to the outsider. More often than not these declarations appear in the form of statements in annual reports, strategic plans, and in the organization's marketing and public-service documents. What is generally not apparent to the outside observer is the extensive work that went into redefining the organization's mission and objectives. In many instances such activity usually extends over a considerable period of time, with different parts of the agency engaged in the effort. Moreover, as a part of the process, the organization's managers and/or governors may have commissioned need assessments, marketing studies, or other background information searches to establish the direction taken.

However, a key feature of redeveloping the organization's goals to reflect a new intercultural orientation is that the directives cannot be left as mere statements. They must be translated into measurable objectives with definite expected outcomes relative to the targeting of specific ethnic populations and developing an overall multicultural readiness.

BUDGET AND RESOURCE ALLOCATION SUPPORT

The redirection of the organization's intercultural goals must also be accompanied by budgetary support and the internal reallocation of organizational resources. This involves delineating in the budget process how the new bilingual/bicultural staff and/or the bicultural-pairs will be supported. If training or consultation assistance is to be required, these personnel areas likewise need budgetary attention. Internal resource allocation will need to be done. All aspects of the organization's redirection of goals to reflect its intercultural orientation will not require new supportive funds. The above-noted internal reallocation of staffing responsibilities could take care of some portions of the proposed, or already ongoing, effort. Some of the cross-cultural upgrading activity could also come in the form of volunteer support from the community, or from other organizations.

However, two caveats must be stated. First, the dementia-care organization cannot depend on the integration of cultural competency at all its personnel and operational levels to just "happen" through the good intentions of all concerned. Second, the overall effort cannot depend solely on volunteers and the goodwill of the target ethnic community. Real funds and real resources must be provided, just as for any other aspect of organizational expertise related to the provision of dementia care.

COMMITMENT TO A PRESENCE IN THE ETHNIC COMMUNITY

In redesigning itself to encompass intercultural capabilities, the organization must also commit to a steady presence in the target ethnic group community or communities (Valle, 1989). The dementia clinic, residential care setting, day care program, or research headquarters may not be physically able to be moved to the locales where the target ethnic groups reside. However, the organization must consider ways to register its presence in the community. For example, the dementia-care organization needs to consider assigning personnel to serve as its representatives or liaisons. The organization likewise can consider establishing a branch near or in the community being targeted for services. In addition, the organization can establish procedures for working directly in the target ethnic group's locale by means of participating in such activities as health fairs or other community events where the dementia-care agency can establish ongoing visibility for itself.

Transfer of Dementia-Care Technology

Another component of the community side of the intercultural engagement effort is the commitment of the dementia-care organization to transfer dementia-care knowledge and technology to the ethnic community being targeted for services. There are four components to this transfer process (Anrow Sciences of Mandex, Inc., 1987). The transfer of technology first takes place in the direct provision of dementia case knowledge and skills through the community-based and indigenous agency infrastructure. As has been indicated before in the discussion, the attention of many community-based organizations serving the target ethnic group will be focused on problems and needs different than dementing illness. Except perhaps in those ethnically diverse communities where an indigenous network of long-term care services has been generated, the attention of many ethnic groups is on other kinds of health problems. Therefore, the dementia-care organization coming into the community must bring its own expertise in an application-ready format.

The second point at which a transfer of technology occurs is when the agency forms bicultural-pairs. The assumption made earlier is that the bicultural member of the pair will be knowledgeable about the ethnic group culture but less knowledgeable in the area of dementing illness. The organization will there-fore need to make provisions to upgrade the dementing illness knowledge and skills of this member of the team.

The third aspect of the transfer of technology is the expectation that the dementia-care organization will be prepared to provide information to the family members themselves (Brownlee, 1978). This is actually a normal part of dementia-care organizational activity. Whenever a dementing illness diagnostic clinic provides information to the caregivers of a dementia-affected patient, a transfer takes place. The same can be said for dementia research, residential care, educational, and community-based settings. The difference is that the transfer of information must be cast in culturally and linguistically compatible formats. The issues and processes involved were already noted in Chapter 3 with regard to communicational exchanges in which messages are able to be encoded and decoded in the context of the target ethnic audience receiving the message. They are also discussed in Chapter 12 with reference to the manner in which information is transculturated for the ethnic group to which it is directed.

The final step in the transfer of technology process is actually back to organization itself. In this context the dementia-care organization, through its staff, gains important knowledge and skill with regard to working in culturally appropriate ways with the target ethnic group clients. In essence, the organization adds to its own service capabilities, picking up additional expertise in working with the ethnic group's clients.

ONGOING SELF-MONITORING AND EVALUATION

A final aspect of the dementia-care organization's ability to expand its intercultural competency is to design and implement ongoing self-monitoring evaluation processes (*Multicultural Outreach Program Manual,* 1994, 4.11). Cross-cultural competency is not to be measured only by the numbers of ethnically diverse clients enrolled, or of the number of staff members employed. Certainly these will be crucial indicators; however, the complete spectrum of organizational intercultural competency-building and service implementation efforts will need to be included in the monitoring process. Most organizations have internal as well as external evaluation procedures and requirements within which cross-cultural competency assessments can be incorporated. These internal evaluation techniques can range from performance evaluations of individual staff through the assessment of how the intercultural engagement goals in the strategic plan have been put into operation. The internal assessment process can also undertake client outcome and impact evaluations. From the external evaluative perspective, it is recognized that dementia-care organizations will be subject to different regulatory demands. For example, some settings, such as skilled nursing facilities, will be assessed under federal regulatory policy as administered through state health departments. Residential settings will meet a different set of regulations through other state departments. Social day care centers and adult day health settings will have their own regulatory auspices. Those health organizations that are registered with the Joint Commission on the Accreditation of Healthcare Organizations will have still other evaluative demands. The list could go on. The issue will be for the dementia-care organization to accommodate the ethnocultural competency evaluative effort to these regulatory processes.

In practice, this should not be as difficult as it might seem. A review of existing regulations indicates that the cultural aspects of the regulations remain a peripheral concern. Therefore, the dementia-care organization that takes on a self-evaluative effort with regard to its intercultural engagement performance will probably make a greater contribution to the development of intercultural competency assessment than is required by present regulatory standards. In this context, the organizational efforts may have actual impact within the field of cross-cultural dementia care, which currently lacks definition and which this text is addressing.

ORGANIZATIONAL INTERCULTURAL ENGAGEMENT: A SUMMARY

There are a number of working principles that can assist the directors of a dementia-care organization when they are considering an overall strategy for implementing an intercultural competency-enhancement effort.

1. **The directors of the organization need to consider an *infusion* rather than an additive strategy.** Intercultural capabilities stand a better chance of flourishing when they are incorporated into the organization's overall internal development plan rather than when they are treated as an added, and occasional ad hoc, effort that is seeking only to meet temporary needs or demands from the community. Dementia-care organizations do not usually put off incorporating new findings about Alzheimer's disease or related dementing illness into their programs, nor do they wait indefinitely to use promising new dementia-care strategies. These are usually quickly integrated into the organization's informational and service repertoires. Cross-cultural knowledge and skills must be handled in the same manner. Instead of waiting for an annual meeting, the quarterly report, or the occasional organizational newsletters, intercultural practice information must be put directly into the organization's formal and informal communication channels at the earliest possible moment. This integration must be done on an ongoing basis. Additive strategies leave vital, culturally relevant information constantly at the outside edge of organizational functions. Additive approaches communicate that intercultural work is less valued than "mainstream" work. In contrast, the steady

integration–infusion approach gives culturally relevant knowledge a timely and appropriate level of recognition.

> Case 10.2a. The dementia-care organization's educational component had developed information packets that were very well received by the several Asian American groups targeted, with whom the materials had been test marketed. The content had been prepared in both print and videotape formats. The comments received made note of the fact that the materials were linguistically and culturally appropriate to each of the different ethnic groups included: Japanese, Chinese, Vietnamese, and so on. Immediately after the materials were completed, the organization began making use of them as an integral part of its ethnically diverse client service activity. All staff, including the monolingual English-speakers, were instructed in the use of the content.

2. **The directors of the organization need to focus on a systems-wide approach rather than on the renovation of a single program or division.** It does happen that advances in cross-cultural activities are made in distinct parts of the organization. For example, the governing board may make a breakthrough in community relations. The line staff may find a way to include a specific ethnic group that had previously been absent from the agency's service roster. In each instance, the gains made—and the innovations in cross-cultural care that are implemented—might reach no farther than the board committee that made the breakthrough or the staff unit that undertook the task of working directly with the ethnically diverse target client members. The organization as a whole may be relatively unaware of what is occurring. Therefore, the organization's directors and managers have to be alert to the agencywide, and even communitywide, importance of what has been developed. The progress made has to be examined for its importance to the organization as a whole. The dementia-care organization cannot afford to leave the new ideas locked into any single personnel level any more than new information about dementing illness can be left in isolation.

> Case 10.2b. The dementia-care organization that had prepared the multi-ethnic Asian American dementia-relevant materials went several steps farther with the implementation of the materials' use. First the materials were made available for use by the agency's bicultural-pairs in their outreach work to families. Second, the materials were also immediately made available to other agencies within the dementia-care organization's service catchment area. Third, the multicultural Asian American materials were presented at several workshops and to the local agency's parent organization at its annual conference.

3. **For the organization to acquire intercultural competency and credibility, the effort must be actual rather than symbolic.** What can occur is that the intercultural innovation that is launched, or the program that is successful, can receive a great deal of immediate recognition. However, this attention may be restricted to publicity or marketing purposes only and not be incorporated into the organization's ongoing activities.

Case 10.3. The dementia-care organization had worked hard at developing the multi-cultural component of its overall strategic plan. The effort had not only been allocated to a strong and persistent subcommittee of equal rank with all the other goals subcommittees, but also had received the concerted attention of the full planning task force throughout the year-long strategic planning effort. However, 2 years into the implementation of the plan itself, the organization's intercultural engagement efforts still remained at the discussion stage. Very few operational objectives had been developed to bring the organization's intercultural efforts abreast of what had originally been intended, let alone had any action been taken.

4. **There must be rewards and incentives for the organization to make the intercultural-capability–building effort an integral part of the organization.** The effort must bring some benefits to both the initiators and the implementers of the cross-cultural capability-enhancement process. Organizations generally have a number of commonly used mechanisms to provide such benefits. These can take the form of monetary incentives, special recognition, or status changes that would accrue to the people who enhance the dementia-care organization's ability to serve ethnically diverse populations.

> Case 10.4. The dementia multicultural group had been very effective in reaching out to a number of specific ethnic groups within the service region. Some of the activity among the Latinos and some portions of the Japanese and Korean Asian American communities had been quite effective in making inroads into these populations. The effort, however, had proceeded much more slowly with regard to the African American and the urban American Indian/Native American groups. Although the staff responsible for the overall effort felt uncomfortable with the differential returns, the project supervisor saw that all of the various outreach coordinators received equal recognition for their time and effort, both in public and in the merit increases provided at the end of the year, regardless of whether all had obtained equal results.

5. **Intercultural capability building is an ongoing process that needs to be modified over time.** Important events can occur. Staffing patterns can change. The ethnic groups themselves may undergo acculturation experiences. The organization must be ready to modify its approaches over time.

> Case 10.5. The organization had worked very diligently to include Latinos into its diagnostic workups relative to dementing illness. This had gone on over a period of several years. However, changes had taken place in the neighborhoods targeted for services. The original Mexican-heritage Hispanic group seemed now to be the minority ethnic subgroup. Many Latinos of Central American background had moved into the area. Among the shifts that had taken place was the fact that the Central American Latino group was of much younger age and was less focused on dementing illness. Only recently were some of the older relatives joining the families here in the United States. Very few families were coming forward to make use of the dementing illness diagnostic and treatment program.

The outreach staff had likewise changed over time. Just one member of the original three practitioners was still with the dementia-care agency. The remaining outreach team member had brought all the changes that had taken place to the attention of her supervisors. However, the organization's managers had been busy with other priorities. The outreach practitioner's reports seemed to go unnoticed, and she felt demoralized.

END NOTE

The development of cross-cultural capabilities within the total dementia-care organization accomplishes two major objectives. First, it positions the organization appropriately with reference to the ethnically diverse social environment. Second, crucial support is provided to the line staff already engaged in service to ethnic group clients. As discussed, the development of organizationwide cross-cultural readiness is a multifaceted undertaking. There are not only many personnel levels to mobilize for the effort, but there also are changes that need to be effected with regard to organizational goals, internal resource distribution, the overall self-monitoring processes, and the flexibility to accommodate changes in the catchment area. However, if properly planned and sequenced, the undertaking need not be overtaxing to the organization as a whole. Moreover, the organization's managers and directors can often call on both internal experts and knowledgeable people from the ethnically diverse groups being targeted for dementia-care services for assistance and consultation with the planned effort. In this manner, the organization moves to what R. R. Thomas (1994) calls going beyond affirmative action and affirming diversity.

Chapter 11

Locating and Working with Cultural Brokers

Cultural brokers have been mentioned throughout the discussion. In the broadest context a cultural broker includes individuals who are able to bridge their own to another's culture. They are part of what Birkel and Reppucci (1983, p. 187) note as open networks that provide connections to other social systems. In this context, cultural brokers represent individuals who can establish working linkages between specifically targeted ethnically diverse populations and dementia-care practitioners and their parent organizations (Valle, 1981; Valle & Bensussen, 1986; Vega & Murphy, 1990). In this format cultural brokers can assist the practitioner and the organization to extend their collective service reach to ethnically diverse groups (Henderson, 1990a, 1990b; L. Mendoza, 1980, 1981a, 1981b; Valle, 1980a, 1988–1989, 1992a; Valle & Bensussen, 1986; Valle & Martinez, 1985). In their most specific role, cultural brokers have been identified as the ethnically diverse member of a bicultural-pair. Here the monocultural English-speaking professional or provider and the bilingual/bicultural broker individual team up to provide direct services to targeted ethnic group client families coming for dementia-related services. Cultural brokers can also serve as knowledgeable key informants, and in this capacity they can assist the practitioner in becoming more knowledgeable about the cultural–historical aspects of the ethnically diverse community. They can also help the organization with its internal intercultural training efforts.

This segment of the discussion will explore all the different aspects of the cultural broker, or ethnic confidant (Brownlee, 1978, p. 10), role with respect to enhancing the dementia-care cultural mapping/intercultural engagement process. Specifically, the discussion will center around: (a) the strategic importance of cultural brokers in the dementia-care arena, (b) techniques for identifying brokers within the target community, (c) approaches to linking to these people, and (d) ways to maintain and reinforce long-term relationships with the cultural brokers at different levels of the organization.

STRATEGIC IMPORTANCE OF A CULTURAL BROKER

As noted at the onset of the overall discussion, the expected growth of ethnically diverse elderly populations will most likely outpace the availability of sufficient bilingual/bicultural practitioners to meet the emergent needs, especially in the area of dementing illness. It is equally unlikely that the ethnic groups by themselves will be able to produce sufficient dementia-capable practitioners to staff the formal care systems involved in the dementing illness arena. Instead, it would appear that the needs of ethnically diverse populations will in all likelihood outstrip the availability of dementia-capable personnel from the mainstream culture and those who are indigenous to the various ethnically diverse cultures.

It is in the capacity of additional, ethnically attuned, personnel that cultural brokers can come to play an essential function. Basically, they can extend the capabilities of existing dementia-focused services in the several capacities noted above as link persons, adjunct educators, and as the bicultural member of a bicultural-pair. In these several roles, the heretofore culturally isolated practitioner and parent organization alike can establish working intercultural connections with the ethnic group being targeted for services (Anrow Sciences of Mandex, Inc., 1987; Brownlee, 1978). It is possible that there may be medical breakthroughs with regard to the early diagnosis of such diseases as Alzheimer's, which accounts for the major portion of late-onset dementia. There may also be breakthroughs in the actual treatment of dementing conditions, either by arresting the symptoms or even by postponing the degenerative processes. However, should any of these advances occur, dementia-care organizations will still be faced with people affected by dementing illness whose course can extend over a 20-year period.

Moreover, as the past history indicates, even if these advances happen it is highly unlikely that the more isolated sectors of the ethnically diverse groups will be early beneficiaries of the technical and medical advances to come. Costs, language barriers, and the fact that many ethnically diverse groups remain outside of the standard routes whereby current Alzheimer's disease and related dementia information is communicated are collectively certain to impede the ethnic group members' access to the discoveries that will be made. Here again, cultural brokers can be mobilized to assist in the processes of disseminating the information about the advances in diagnosis and treatment that might be made. More important, the cultural brokers can assist ethnically diverse populations in accessing dementia-care practitioners and their parent organizations

Cultural brokers are not being proposed as a panacea for ethnically diverse populations to access dementia-care services; rather, they function as a supportive strategy. They can be considered a form of "supplemental service coverage capability" for the ethnically diverse community. Moreover, cultural brokers are not being offered as resources to be exploited. Established dementia-care organizations will need to find monetary and other ways to compensate for the cultural brokers for their time and effort. In addition, as presented in Chapters 8 and 9, it is still incumbent on mainstream culture professionals and providers, as well as on their service organizations, to acquire the intercultural capabilities inherent in being able to work in the multicultural environment. The requirement on the part of both practitioners and their parent organizations to attain cultural mapping/intercultural competency remains in place.

IDENTIFYING CULTURAL BROKERS

Cultural brokers can literally range from non-degreed community volunteers and community aides to practitioners with advanced degrees who remain active in the target ethnically diverse community. Cultural brokers can therefore include professionals and providers already working in dementia-care settings. Many bilingual/bicultural practitioners already play this role within their parent systems. However, for purposes of the discussion, it would be better to consider cultural brokers apart from the paid professionals or providers who have the central service responsibility for specific ethnocultural clients within their current organizations. The fact that such individuals are present within their own settings is important, but the cultural broker role must also be examined in a broader perspective.

It should be noted that cultural brokers can also come from the dementia-affected families themselves. Warnings about the proper uses of such individuals as go-betweens have been outlined in Chapter 5 and other parts of the discussion. The issue noted earlier is to avoid putting family members into conflictual situations by asking them to side with both the external dementia-care organization and the family's interests. If these aspects of the agency–family go-between are kept in mind, the idea of a family cultural broker has considerable merit. This individual can function as a built-in intercultural communicator as well as an in-house assistant relative to meeting the care-giving needs of the dementia-affected family member.

The literature sees cultural brokers as exemplifying a number of identifiable characteristics (Lubben, 1988; Mendoza, 1980, 1981b; Smith, 1975; Valle, 1980a; Valle & Bensussen, 1986; Vega & Murphy, 1990), applicable also to the field of dementia (Valle, 1988–1989). These features include: (a) having bilingual and bicultural capabilities relative to the their specific ethnic group; (b) being already identified somewhere in the community, often by word-of-mouth, as a helper/broker; (c) maintaining a demonstrated ethnic-community–focused career track over time; and (d) maintaining the capability of adapting to many different situations as well as working with a wide range of people and systems. The range of characteristics by which cultural brokers can be identified is summarized in Box 11.1.

It should be noted that many cultural brokers meeting the above profile character-

Communicational/Interactional Capabilities
- Maintains bilingual/bicultural communications capabilities from native language to mainstream culture.
- Is a central person relative to indigenous clients and the mainstream contacts. Is very people-interaction oriented.
- Can work with a wide range of people of different statuses.
- Does not attempt to polarize communicational situations.
- Is often known by word-of-mouth reputation but can also be identified by the frequency of contacts with different organizations or agencies when bringing indigenous clients or seeking to locate resources.
- Knows the cultural protocols for establishing trust and rapport not only in own culture of origin but also with regard to the mainstream culture.

Indigenous Career Emphasis/Systemic Considerations
- Is service- and resource-distribution–oriented in contrast to engaging in "political" and "influence" exchanges. The practitioner–cultural broker link is best maintained when the focus is service oriented and when the transfer of skills and knowledge takes place. The broker will engage in advocacy, but this is client-focused advocacy. The broker usually will not be found among the community's "leaders." The broker will be out performing services.
- Has an identified career track or specialty practice or natural/indigenous helping activity; some can be indigenous counselors, healers, community organizers. Practitioners need to identify the broker's specialty area to make most appropriate use of natural expertise.
- Knows resources and their uses and is constantly trying to update/upgrade information about them.
- Can adapt to many different circumstances and situations.
- There can be multiple cultural brokers, with different indigenous career specialty backgrounds in any given ethnically diverse community.

Special Features and Considerations
- There can be specific family brokers or go-betweens. However these brokers should not be given double duty to be loyal to the family and act as pseudopractitioners.
- Professionals and practitioners who are indigenous to the ethnic culture being targeted for services can also take on a cultural broker role.

Box 11.1   Cultural broker profile.

istics can be found within any given geographic area as well as within any one ethnocultural group. However, the professional or provider must be aware that all of the cultural brokers who are located will not necessarily know each other. Some will know one another, but most will be carrying out their own cultural linking responsibilities. This means, therefore, that there are not indigenous organizations of cultural brokers; rather, it is best if they are seen as linkpersons who fall into a structural niche between indigenously organized groups such as ethnic clubs or associations and the dementia-affected ethnic family groups. They are also in between the community and the external formal organizational systems such as dementia-care agencies. In fact, Brownlee (1978, pp. 8–11) distinguishes between "community confidants" (brokers) and "community leaders." Figure 11.1 highlights the linkperson pivotal position of the cultural broker.

For dementia-care purposes, it is important to regard the cultural broker as a linkperson rather than as a representative of an organized group, otherwise the professional or provider will be disappointed when a broker is mobilized for a dementia-

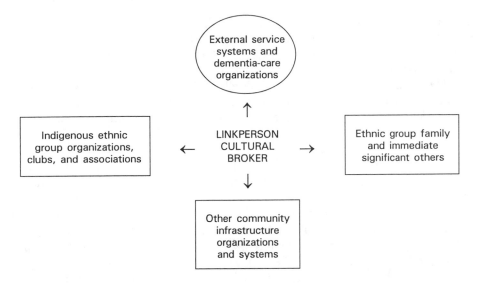

Figure 11.1   Cultural broker as a linkperson.

related service and does not come forward with an additional group of indigenous helpers. He or she may know other brokers and share insights and information, but again, for the most part the cultural brokers at the local community level go about their duties independently of each other. Moreover, they do not represent a social movement in the usual, more "political" sense of the idea, that is, they may know about the political processes in the ethnic community, but they do not function as the community's leaders. Box 11.2 can perhaps help clarify this important notion. The

SERVICE AND RESOURCE DISTRIBUTION NETWORKS	POWER AND INFLUENCE NETWORKS
*Cultural rapport and trust orientations predominate	*Resource acquisition and decision making control focus predominates
*Indigenous helping career tracks are followed	*Indigenous leadership roles/relationships are implemented
*Cultural broker is usually less visible to the cultural outsider; is identified through cultural pathways	*Influence broker is usually visible to the cultural outsider; is identified through power/influence networks

- Both types of indigenous brokers play useful *but distinct* roles within the ethnically diverse community.
- Some cultural brokers can have a role in both types of indigenous networks. However, when working with clients in need; and specifically dementia-affected indigenous clients, cultural brokers will remain service focused. They will *not* engage in power and influence behaviors.

Box 11.2   Service orientation of the cultural broker.

cultural brokers in most ethnically diverse cultures fill the niche of indigenously assisting individuals and families with their self-acquired or, better put, culturally acquired problem-solving and service-resource–linking skills. The cultural brokers will fit the service and resource distribution side of Box 11.2.

The distinction between the cultural brokers' linking functions in contrast to attributing "political" influence is an important consideration for practitioners and their parent organizations. First, if the professional or provider, or the dementia-care organization, wants to locate the appropriate type of cultural broker, he or she will need to look in the service sector of the ethnic community rather than in its leadership circles. Other types of brokers are active in the latter arena. Second, the cultural brokers will feel misused if they are taken from their more customary service-related roles. Third, the organization will stand to lose the broker–agency linkage if the broker determines that the dementia-care organization is acting from political rather than service-directed objectives. Cultural brokers are not naive with regard to their own community and the external community; rather, their goals are directed toward providing services. Also, as noted earlier, it is important to remember that, when initially contacted, cultural brokers will only rarely be dementia specialists. They can develop these skills and take on the dementing-care service responsibilities. Perhaps, as the ties between dementia-care oriented practitioners and cultural brokers expand, more dementia-knowledgeable brokers will surface. However, for the present, when community brokers are encountered they will not necessarily be working on Alzheimer's disease and related disorder concerns. In assuming the capacity of the agency link-person, adjunct trainer, or bicultural-pair team member, the nature of their community roles makes them quick learners of new areas of services to bring to the community, such as dementia care. At the same time it should not be forgotten that the cultural brokers are coming from a people-oriented perspective, and their strengths should not be diverted to performing bureaucratic-type tasks to serve other organizational purposes.

Case 11.1. The dementia-care program had determined to engage a large and underserved Latino community population within the agency's catchment area. The program manager was concerned that, even though some outreach had been attempted in the past, including the distribution of information to the community, few family members and patients had yet come forward. The manager decided on another approach. A bilingual/bicultural Latino outreach team was formed. It included two monocultural English-speaking staff who were dementia specialists and a part-time Latina consultant who was working on her master's degree. The consultant knew the target community as she had been volunteering her time at a health clinic. She welcomed the new paid position. She also welcomed the opportunity to learn about dementing illness. The outreach team began to operate in the target community, contacting families almost immediately as the consultant picked up on dementing illness right away. However, difficulties arose when the organization's managers recognized the cultural-broker consultant's people skills and began diverting her activities to improving the agency's position in the community. The cultural broker found more of her time filled with attending meetings and giving talks to important organizations in the community. Shortly thereafter she left her position and returned to her health clinic volunteer role.

By formally taking on a bicultural staff member, as illustrated in Case 11.1, the organization sent a positive signal to the ethically diverse community. It seemed that the bicultural team would work out. However, troubles came when the cultural broker was given assignments that took her away from what she felt comfortable doing and put her to work in an area she did not perceive as service oriented.

Finally, in identifying cultural brokers as in all other aspects of the intercultural engagement process, it is important to be alert to the actual ethnic diversity within the community. For example, Haitians may be phenotypically similar to African Americans, but they are culturally and linguistically distinct. The search for cultural brokers has to be undertaken with ethnic group heterogeneity in mind.

Case 11.2. The dementia-care organization had developed a good working relationship with the African American community within its service catchment. The organization's service coordinator, an African American professional, wanted now to reach out to the Haitian American community but knew that the organization could not proceed until a Haitian-speaking linkperson who was familar with the target ethnic group and its language could be located. He proceeded to review the organization's service records and identified a nurse from a Haitian community clinic who had called on occasion to ask about dementing illness issues. Through her help two additional interested volunteers were eventually located, and a beginning outreach plan to the Haitian ethnic group was initiated.

Recognizing the need to tap into culturally appropriate networks, the coordinator in Case 11.2, who was quite familiar with the African American community, applied his expertise to start the linking process to an entirely different ethnocultural group.

LINKING TO THE CULTURAL BROKERS

Linking to the cultural brokers involves several actions (Valle, 1980a, 1988–1989). Some of the approaches have already been noted in the cases discussed above and mentioned elsewhere throughout the narrative, including Chapter 9. As a summary of the processes involved, in initiating the linkage the practitioner must: (a) be familiar with the target ethnic group's culture and its local history, (b) be able to apply community observation skills, (c) maintain an active presence in the community, (d) include ongoing networking with the target ethnic community's own indigenous organizations as a part of the linking activity, and (e) develop a pattern of consistency in the messages communicated to the target ethnic community groups as well as a consistency in following through with promised actions or assigned tasks.

Familiarity with the Cultural Group

To initiate the broker linkage-outreach effort, professionals and providers must familiarize themselves with the target ethnic community, as outlined in Part One and specifically in Chapter 3. It is true that one cannot fully get to know the designated ethnic community through external records, particularly as in each regional setting the ethnic group members develop their own interactional flavor. However, initial preparation can bring potential brokers to the surface. This activity can take the form of reviewing records and reports about the community, or looking over one's own home organization's records, along with actually engaging the community either in person or by telephone. In Case 11.2, the African American practitioner reviewed the dementia-care organizations' own records. It was clear to the practitioner that the community health clinic nurse would be the key person through whom to initiate the contact to a new ethnic group.

However, in following through with the methodology of gaining familiarity with the target ethnic group, the practitioner has to change focus. In the search for cultural brokers the professional or provider moves from a micro, or family perspective, to a macro orientation. In this context the target ethnocultural community processes are viewed from a more comprehensive vantage point. This means finding ways to understand the pulse of the daily life of the target ethnic community from a service delivery standpoint as well as getting to know the preferred pathways that the members of the ethnic group use to get to and from the services they need. Case 11.2 is too sketchily drawn to provide the full impact of the different perspective taken by the dementia-care services coordinator to locate cultural brokers and to locate family members for the program. With regard to the brokers, the professionals or providers must apply a community-systems analysis approach, which enables them to see who is helping, not just who is in need.

In the process of becoming familiar with the target ethnic community to get to know its cultural brokers, the practitioner can gain the assistance of the initial links who might have been located to serve as informal instructors from the cultural group. These broker–teachers can in turn be put to use to link further into the ethnic community. What the professional or provider does is assemble and organize all the content received, in whatever form the information is given. This information is then sifted through to develop a working profile of the interactive *people systems* that are active within the target ethnocultural group locale.

Broker-Focused Guided Observation Techniques

Carefully directed observations of the community processes can greatly facilitate the process of identification of the presence of cultural brokers. Here the professional or provider looks to see who might fit the profile of a cultural broker. Although no one broker will have all of the characteristics displayed in Box 11.1, most will demonstrate features of each of the principal categories. By the application of cultural mapping techniques, now focused at the macro level of community life, the professional's or provider's interculturally attuned cultural eyes and ears can generally begin to identify potential brokers.

Case 11.3. The practitioner had purposely been searching for several cultural brokers to assist in the dementing illness outreach effort to the Latino community. He had begun to hear several names repeatedly mentioned in a helping context, although none seemed related to dementia service. They included a Mrs. Acuña, a Mr. Garcia, and a Mrs. Jacobs, all bilingual Spanish-speakers and known to volunteer to help seniors. He had also checked out the fact that all three persons appeared in the agency's records as referring several families for assistance, which also served as a backup insight to their being potential brokers.

Given these leads, the practitioner followed up to see and directly contact these three potential candidates for cultural brokers. In making the observational rounds of the community processes, it is important to steer away from stereotypes such as surnames. In the present era of interethnic marriage and cross-cultural contact, a potential broker could have a surname that sounds like it is from the mainstream cultural group, but could very well be interculturally connected with the target ethnic community. In the search for cultural brokers the practitioner also needs to go beyond surface characteristics and determine if the potential candidate meets the criteria of the cultural broker profile in the actual context of community activity and service and, most important, whether the cultural broker candidate is able and willing, or is actually suited, to work in the dementia-care arena.

The practitioner actually engages in a process that involves identification of potential candidates, direct interaction with them, and negotiations about the work that is involved. Things cannot be left to chance. The potential gains for the dementia-care organization, the practitioner, the cultural broker, and the ethnically diverse community have to be discussed openly—not always in a business manner, but in a culturally sensitive realistic format. Whenver possible, cultural brokers need to receive some form of compensation, which can come in the form of a consultancy, reimbursement for travel and meals, or other possible types of recognition available at the organization; for example, certificates acknowledging the broker's services, or credit for the work done if the broker is in some school program. Obviously, the different types of formal recognition can be used in combination.

A very strong motivator thatcultural brokers bring to their activity is an altruistic or helping orientation (Valle & Mendoza, 1978, p. 69). The issue for the professional or provider, or the parent dementia care organization, seeking to make the connection with cultural brokers, is not to take advantage of this very powerful drive found among people who opt for cultural broker roles. The rubric of cultural reciprocity and mutualism, spoken of in Chapter 5, mandates that the practitioner and agency return something to the ethnocultural community and its cultural brokers.

Continuing Presence in the Community

A process that greatly facilitates locating and linking to cultural brokers is to have the professional or provider maintain a continuing presence in the community. The visibility to be gained for the practitioner's and their parent organization is invaluable. Basically, this means attending local coordinating council-type meetings; making presentations to community groups, including both provider and community-based groups; and being on the other end of countless telephone contacts and inquiries or, as noted earlier in the discussion, just being present on festive occasions.

From an organizational standpoint this type of effort may appear too labor intensive, involving considerable outlay of time and effort. However, it is crucial that the practitioner and the organization continue to stay with the interpersonal contact activity throughout the total process. In the early stages of the effort, when the initial broker and community contacts are being made, the interpersonal engagement effort is especially crucial. All of the different contacts are really evaluating whether the community should "do business" with the professional or provider and the organization. In the later stages, when the linkages and contacts have turned to mutual interest and a mutual-trust arrangement, the interpersonal contacts and linkages are equally vital. In these phases the professional or provider, or parent organization, is presenting direct proof of the consistency of their commitment.

Nonetheless, the overall undertaking may appear as "too much" effort expended for the amount of first returns obtained. Even experienced intercultural practitioners will at times question their own investment of time and effort. However, it must be kept in mind that many ethnically diverse groups may not have received the best treatment at the hands of prior practitioners or organizations with similar missions. Present good intentions are not enough. The status that professionals and providers enjoy in their own circles does not necessarily carry over to the ethnoculturally diverse environment. That status has to be earned. Moreover, the organizations active in the target ethnic community feel some responsibility to protect their needy family members, especially the elderly. The professional's or provider's demonstrated willingness to go through the ongoing "screening" process conducted by all the people who are engaged will go a long way toward establishing the practitioner's and the parent organization's community credentials.

Consistency Over Time

When engaging the ethnic community's organizational infrastructure and its indigenous cultural brokers, the practitioner must remain consistent over time. Relational ties and services cannot be turned on and off. If cutbacks are expected, or if the professional or provider's organization has specific time, resource, or eligibility limitations, these need to be stated up front. If the practitioner makes a service offer or accepts a specific responsibility, the effort needs to be carried out and the responsibility fulfilled. It can happen that unexpected events will change the practitioner's plans. In such instances frankness about the inability to follow through has to be reported openly and directly. It will be very devastating to both the practitioner and to the community if the effort is tagged with negative impressions, even if this happens inadvertently.

It is true that in the present climate of funding for services many service organizations are undergoing dramatic changes. This is particularly so in the health services arena, where the practitioner roles, responsibilities, the underlying ownership of a program or organization can change overnight. Funding for a specific aspect of agency function may be eliminated. In such circumstances, staff may be discharged, or the original mission of the organization may be discarded and a new one substituted. All of these factors can generate major difficulties for the professional or provider seeking to establish a stable relationship with a particular ethnocultural community. However, in intercultural engagement practice, it is crucial to see the issues from the perspective of the target ethnocultural group members.

The likelihood is that individual ethnic group members and the organizations indigenous to the community will have been down this path before. Professionals and providers have come and gone without fulfilling the originally proposed efforts. Anything from barriers to eligibility to the failure on the part of the practitioner to gain true cultural understanding may have severed the intended pattern. Hence, the new practitioner entering the interethnic scene may find initial reluctance on the part of the ethnic community members to participate. The expectations of the ethnocultural group members may be low. They may be holding back their participation to see if the professionals or providers hold up their end of the intended effort.

Consistency over time by the practitioner and the parent dementia-care organization can do much to overcome the residual effects of the types of previous experiences and failed expectations just mentioned. In this context, therefore, the parent organization's managers as well as the practitioners themselves must look ahead to when either a specific individual, engaged in the ethnocultural community interaction, will be assigned different duties or will go on extended leave. Every effort should be made to inform the key community network actors when changes in the continuous presence over time by the professional or provider will occur. Wherever possible a backup contact and community engagement support plan need to be put into place.

As difficult, and even sidetracking from the main dementia-service goal as these community engagement efforts may seem, the contacts will bear fruit. Through consistency of effort over time the professionals and providers can move from being observers only to becoming active players in the community processes. Moreover, an active presence in the target ethnic community will often yield valuable insights into how to better shape the dementia-service engagement process with the target ethnic client group as well as to how to strengthen the linkages to the ethnic group's cultural brokers.

In essence, an ethnocultural broker outreach effort, once begun, must be ready to continue over the long run. However, everything cannot be expected to go smoothly every time, and the professional or provider may have to improvise

Case 11.4. The initial cultural brokers who had been contacted to connect to the community had not come through. Other service concerns seemed to be given priority consideration over dementing illness issues. The dementia needs assessment project coordinator himself, not an African American, decided to take another approach. He sought out an African American colleague in another city with community-outreach capabilities. The project coordinator was invited to fly into the city the following week to meet and work out the details of the dementia needs assessment among African Americans.

At the meeting seven volunteers, in addition to the faculty colleague and her mother, were present. All were hired for the dementia-assessment project based on the colleague's reputation as a people-finder and an initial training session was held. The community-outreach colleague became the supervisor at the new site and the dementia assessment project coordinator agreed to fly in monthly for in-person reviews of progress. In the interim, phones and electronic mail would be used for communications. The outreach team fanned out through their own networks, and within 3 short weeks had located enough dementia-affected caregivers in the African American community to make a substantive contribution to the overall findings of the community-needs assessment.

One cannot always contact the right brokers. Often, community needs and the priorities do not coincide with the intended outreach effort. Moreover, everything cannot be done on a volunteer basis; there are times when one has to pay consultant fees. However, persistent networking and searching for the right mix of cultural brokers within the target ethnic group can eventually produce positive results.

OVERVIEW OF CULTURAL BROKER ROLES

Cultural brokers can play a variety of roles relative to the target ethnocultural community. For example, some will be seen as providing indigenous information and referral services, and others will be engaged in offering specific types of services that may range from indigenous counseling through community advocacy assistance (Mendoza, 1981a). Still others will provide more concrete assistance, such as transportation. Some will have broad spheres of activities and be able to work with a wide range of systems, whereas still other brokers will have more circumscribed areas of responsibility. The family cultural brokers spoken of throughout the various parts of the text would fill the latter category. Cultural brokers at this level can relate to outside systems but in a more limited way. In contrast, the cultural brokers identified in the cases described in this chapter would fit the profile of people who can interact with many different kinds of systems outside of their own neighborhoods and immediate ethnocultural communities.

From a more analytical standpoint, some of the literature (Mendoza, 1980, 1981a, 1981b) has referred to cultural brokers as having identifiable career tracks. For example, they may demonstrate a natural helping pattern as counselors or indigenous health practitioners. Others may in effect operate at the community-organization level, assisting their indigenous clienteles to take various actions on their own behalf.

However, it is important to indicate that the professional or provider cannot expect to find formal cultural broker job descriptions out in the community, even in the community-based agencies. Job descriptions for aide-level staff will not work for the task of identifying cultural brokers. These job descriptions are based on a modified professional task model. Individuals from the various ethnically diverse populations to be encountered will simply carry out brokering activity the way they see best. It is the practitioner who must: (a) identify what kind of cultural brokering activity is going on, (b) discover the strengths and limitations of this activity, (c) determine if indeed the individual performing the activity fits the profile of a cultural broker, and (d) find the means to establish working relationships with the potential broker candidates relative to culturally relevant dementia concerns.

Regardless of the level at which they operate and the service approaches that they adopt, an obviously central role that the cultural brokers can play is that of the gatekeepers who can be most helpful in assisting the practitioners, or the dementia-care organizations, to better understand and serve the target ethnocultural group. In addition, for the monocultural, English-speaking, mainstream culture practitioner, cultural brokers become the linchpin of the bicultural-pair. For the already bilingual/ bicultural professional or provider, cultural brokers serve as a means to extend and enhance their intercultural engagement activities within the target ethnic community.

SUMMARY OF BROKER LINKAGE TACTICS AND TECHNIQUES

There are a number of elements to consider in implementing a cultural broker linkage effort. Therefore, to ensure the continuity of the approach, the professional or provider engaged in community outreach to locate and involve cultural brokers outreach needs to proceed as follows.

1. **The practitioner needs to design a long-range cultural broker linkage plan and maintain it in place.** Multicultural engagement and ethnic-specific linkage, especially with the cultural broker, works most effectively to the extent that it is accompanied by a plan to support the effort (Goodman, 1989). Just because the target ethnic community is in need of Alzheimer's disease and related disorders information and service resources does not mean that cultural brokers will be automatically responsive to the dementing illness message. Among many ethnocultural groups, dementing illness emphasis will probably still be new for some period ahead because the group members will often be coming into contact with information on dementia for the first time. Dementia may not even be recognized for what it is until its more advanced stages (Ross et al., 1997).

   Also, it takes time and concerted effort to establish an interactional-communication outreach format. Therefore, both long- and short-term goals are needed to take advantage of the immediate opportunities that present themselves as well as to handle the pauses in community response. The latter may give the appearance that the effort has stalled. A working plan provides direction and assurances to those involved in the activity that they are moving in a well-thought-out direction.

2. **The practitioner must be patient in the short run, because the initial results from all of the linkage efforts may be slow in coming.** Professionals and providers need to become used to being "tested" by the potential community brokers. This is perhaps somewhat troublesome to established professionals and providers, and this experience is especially hard to accept by practitioners who may see the overwhelming needs of the ethnically diverse dementia-affected elder and all of the involved family members/significant others. In the urgencies provoked by the situation, it can appear that the delays are creating additional stressors for the family network. However, the process is akin to consumers responding to new products. Occasionally it takes time to establish the products' viability.

3. **The practitioner needs to be flexible and willing to adapt the original plan to changing circumstances within the target ethnic community.** Needless to say, contingency plans to accompany the main plan to guide the

broker outreach and linkage effort as it actually takes shape are essential. Case 11.4 can serve as an example of a contingency plan being put into effect.

4. **The practitioner must seek to build a community reputation for consistency and aim to develop a word-of-mouth credibility.** Intercultural outreach and linkage works best when the families themselves begin to come forward and communicate with each other about the positive aspects of the services received. As with other aspects of Alzheimer's disease and dementing illness outreach, this step can be attained in the form of caregivers from the target ethnic group and their families who have already been helped and who now want to volunteer to help others. These people acting as cultural brokers often serve best as the word-of-mouth support for the outreach effort. They can also serve as the nuclei of a support group and specific educational outreach activities. In various projects that are undertaken, word-of-mouth has usually been found to begin taking effect around the sixth month of the project and continues in an ascending curve throughout the remainder of the effort, extending beyond the life of a specific program.

It should be noted that word-of-mouth referrals also come from the indigenous aides and formal agency provider sectors. Often these referrals reinforce those made by family members who report positive experiences with the Alzheimer's disease and related dementing illness outreach effort. What is implicit in word-of-mouth credibility is the demonstrated willingness by the practitioner or the parent dementia-care organization to deliver the support and assistance and stand by the ethnocultural community and its members over time.

5. **The practitioner must be willing to monitor the effort on an ongoing basis.** This means that the practitioner and the parent organization must maintain a readiness to evaluate the outcomes and impact of the overall effort. It cannot be expected that everything will work out in a neat and orderly fashion. The practitioner's steadiness of purpose will do much to make the broker linkage and recruitment effort work out.

END NOTE

Cultural brokers can greatly extend the practitioner's and the parent dementia-care organization's cultural mapping/intercultural engagement capabilities. The strategy to locate, link, and involve cultural brokers in service to ethnoculturally diverse populations does take time and effort. From the dementia-care organization's directors' and managers' perspectives, this may appear as the diversion of scarce resources. However, from the standpoint of those with the experience in trying the approach, the outcomes are quite rewarding in several respects. First, the professional or provider finds extra eyes, ears, and hands with which to bring dementia-care resources to previously underserved populations. Second, there is actually a multiplier-type effect. The linkages yield much more in the form of a community presence and credibility than the practitioner's efforts alone would appear to produce. The linkages actually extend on a communitywide basis. Third, from the perspective of the growing need for ethnically competent and dementia-capable personnel, cultural brokers are a potential bright spot. The need for interculturally proficient practitioners can be partially met through this strategy. However, as stated earlier, cultural brokers are not the cure for the interculturally competent dementia service. The organization itself has to be ready to move decisively into the intercultural engagement arena in the manner outlined in Chapter 10.

Chapter 12

Culturally Attuning
the Dementia-Care Message

Much of what is cultural is communicated through language and symbols. Therefore, it is most appropriate that the practitioner and the parent dementia-care organization consider the impact of formal messages disseminated through a wide range of communication channels, including letters to clients, reports, brochures, and the available print, audio, and visual media sources (Alzheimer's Disease and Related Disorders Association, 1994; Braun et al., 1995; Sizemore et al., 1991). The content can range from eligibility criteria, diagnostic results, and treatment plans, as well as a wide range of medical and scientific information about dementing conditions. To be effective, this content must be delivered in *culture-fair* (i.e., linguistically equivalent) formats (Valle, 1989, pp. 123–126, 1994, p. 35). Moreover, for some segments of the ethnically diverse populations the material must also be converted into a *literate-fair* presentation that takes into account the literacy level of the intended audience. The dementia-focused information, if tailored to the culture, language, and literacy level of the target ethnic client group, can provide a powerful support to the overall intercultural exchange process. If poorly prepared and neither culturally nor linguistically attuned, or if it goes beyond the literacy capabilities of the target ethnic group clientele, the information will create major barriers to cross-cultural understanding.

In preparing dementia-related information and delivering it to different ethno-cultural groups, the professional or practitioner uses the same range of intercultural communication–linguistic considerations covered in Chapter 4. Careful attention to all of the nuances involved in encoding and decoding of messages (see Figure 4.1) is required. However, in the present discussion, the focus of the practitioner and the parent dementia-care organization is on the macro level, or ethnic community-wide aspects of intercultural communication. Nonetheless, careful attention, equal to or even exceeding that of interpersonal communications, has to be given to the processes surrounding the assembly and dissemination of messages to culturally diverse groups.

The growing use of automated phone messages with multiple instructions to the caller, as well as the increasing complexity of billing and other processes for consumers, already poses considerable difficulty for ethnic group members who primarily rely on their native language. Therefore, whatever can be done to ease the burden of understanding the messages being communicated to ethnically diverse populations will in turn augment the intercultural engagement process.

The discussion that follows centers around: (a) reviewing the principles underlying the transculturation of messages and communications to ethnically diverse populations and putting them into what can be called culture-fair as well as literate-fair communications (b) delineating the differences between simply translating messages and communications rather than transculturating them, (c) specifying several sets of working principles to facilitate the overall intercultural communication process, and (d) making certain that a dissemination plan accompanies the effort to culturally attune the dementia-care message.

OVERVIEW OF THE ISSUES

Communication with culturally and linguistically diverse groups is becoming ever more important as U.S. society becomes more heterogeneous (Anrow Sciences of Mandex, Inc., 1987). Very often health professionals and human service organizations seeking to communicate with non-English-speaking audiences try to translate their information directly. This can produce several difficulties. First, as was indicated in Chapter 4, the other language may not have equivalent technical terms, that is, the other cultural idiom may use colloquial rather than medical terminology to depict the different dementing disorders. It is not that such terms as *Alzheimer's disease* should be avoided. However, it is vitally important to link to locally used language to facilitate communication of the intended content (Brownlee, 1978) in a culture-fair way.

Second, straight-out translation may bypass the local evolution of the ethnic language, particularly where the target ethnic group has resided in a host society for some time. Therefore, professionals and agencies seeking to communicate with culturally diverse populations need to really get to know colloquial idiom of the target communities. If one wants to communicate about Alzheimer's disease and/or related disorders, there is a need to find out how the other culture thinks and talks about the problem if, for example, the other culture denies or hides dementing conditions, or attaches religious values to them. The scientific message, then, has to be appropriately interwoven into these various different cultural, communicational, and value matrices.

Third, straight-out translation may ignore key sociodemographic factors that may be affecting the target ethnic group population. Agencies seeking to develop informational materials for a specific ethnic group audience may think immediately about obtaining a formal translator. Little thought may be given as to whether the translator knows the sociodemographic and literacy profile of the target audience along with the language. In such instances too much technical jargon can slip into the proposed communication even in its translated form. Moreover, from still another standpoint, if the translator is also less familiar with a particular health field such as Alzheimer's disease and dementing illness, the translated content might emerge in very correct Spanish, Japanese, or any other ethnic group language; however, it may "miss the boat" entirely with regard to communicating to the target group about dementing illness.

TRANSCULTURATION: CLARIFICATION OF TERMS

Before going further in the discussion it might be useful to clarify a number of terms being used relative to designing and implementing communications across cultures. The process of *transculturation* refers to first approaching the information to be communicated from the other culture's viewpoint rather than the mainstream English-speaking cultural framework. Transculturation is actually an extension of many of the cultural mapping/intercultural engagement principles outlined throughout Part One. The professional or provider does not start only with what has to be translated, but rather takes the perspective of how the people from the other culture will think about the information to be provided.

> Case 12.1. The slogan of the Alzheimer's Association, "Someone to Stand by You," can be directly translated into Spanish as *"Alguien a su lado."* However, when the slogan is translated it emerges with quite a different connotation than that originally intended. In English the slogan is clear: There is a reliable, supportive, and caring "someone" available at the caregiver's side, namely, the association itself. In Spanish, instead of a "supportive" someone the direct translation emerges as a "someone" who is there to be "nosy" and/or who is behaving in an "intrusive" manner. The original phrase is really an "Anglicism" idiomatically residual to English. What was needed, therefore, was to transculturate the intended slogan. A more culturally syntonic statement that emerged in the Spanish idiom was *"Alguien con quien contar,"* that is, someone to count on or to rely upon. This latter version also was the slogan actually being used by the Alzheimer's associations in Mexico and Puerto Rico, both of whom had arrived at it independently.

Lack of careful attention to the pitfalls of the literal translation approach can lead to problems with regard to outreach, data gathering, and symptom interpretation communications with culturally diverse populations. The initiation of the transculturation strategy, such as in Case 12.1, creates a more level playing field whereby the professional and provider can move ahead with the already-difficult task of working with families facing dementing illness within their midst.

PRINCIPLES OF TRANSCULTURATING MESSAGES

The *transculturation* process itself can be broken down into a series of working principles. First, it is important to specify the message. There are a multiplicity of messages possible in the dementing illness arena. However, it is important that the professional or provider start with what is intended to be communicated with respect to the specific circumstances facing the ethnically diverse family members or a larger ethnic group target audience. For example, will the message be about the differential diagnostic process itself? Will it be about recognizing the symptoms? Will it be about accessing different kinds of services? Or is the message directed to the caregivers themselves? Thought has to be given to these considerations from the start. If a group of practitioners is to be involved, or if the dementia-care organization as a whole will be involved, discussions along these lines must take place among all the people who will play a role in the intended communication.

Second, depending on the complexity of the message, it has to be partialized. Many health-related messages, however specifically focused, are complex in nature. Alzheimer's disease is especially difficult. For one, it is still diagnosed on the basis of symptoms and by the exclusion of all other possible conditions. In addition, because the assessment of dementing illness usually requires multidisciplinary or multispecialty professional input, there may be many different technical aspects of the message, which in turn need to be communicated. This step is particularly important relative to assisting caregivers and family members to understand the dementing condition and to develop a culturally appropriate careplan.

Third, it is equally important to make a comprehensive assessment of the target audience and its potential or actual familiarity with the intended message. For example, will the present communication be the first one to the family or ethic group members? Have there been prior communications with the target ethnic group? If so, what has been the family's or the group's response? It could be that the ethnic group members have some beginning familiarity with some aspects of the proposed content. It is even possible that the content is generally well known to the ethnic group, but some specific refinements are needed. All of these aspects need to be addressed in the communications assessment phase of transculturation of the intended message. The professional or provider entering the direct intercultural communication situation will often find that the proposed communication will require a unique "slant" to make it culturally-fair relative to the family or larger ethnically diverse group being addressed.

Fourth, the practitioner needs to maintain a balanced perspective. It is important to keep in mind that target audience receptivity is not assured just because there is a well-designed and culturally-fair message at hand. Some type of planned information preparation and dissemination program about dementing illness concerns needs to go hand in hand with any transculturation efforts undertaken to assist ethnically diverse communities and individual families. This can begin with assessments as to the most culturally compatible formats to use. All the tools available to professionals and providers as well as to their parent dementia-care organizations to assess community need can be made culturally appropriate. These can include anything from surveys, through focus groups, to key informants. The application of the cultural–historical information-gathering strategies described in Chapter 3 can likewise be used. At times information relevant to the ethnic group's preferred communication style, or even examples of culturally compatible content, can be located in this manner.

Putting Principles into Action

Putting the transculturation approach into action involves a series of practical steps.

1. **Some form of intercultural communication working group is assembled.** The working group must include people who are (a) fully bicultural and bilingual with respect to the target ethnic audience, (b) knowledgeable about the local/regional idiom and colloquial language usages and, equally important, (c) knowledgeable about Alzheimer's disease and related disorders. With regard to this last point, although it is crucial to convey information in a *culturally compatible* format, the intercultural work group must make certain that the information is accurate with respect to the specific dementing conditions being portrayed. Just because a cultural group holds certain beliefs about the causes of dementing conditions does not mean that the underlying physiological, medical, and scientific facts about such disorders as Alzheimer's disease are to be overlooked or downplayed. Yes, the information must link to the ethnocultural group's language and normative ways of thinking, but it must also represent what is really known about dementing illness.

2. **The intercultural communication group begins to generate the linguistically and culturally appropriate content.** The intercultural communication work group proceeds to develop the necessary content. It can happen that, at the start, the work group will already have some "translated" Alzheimer's disease or other dementing illness content on hand. This material is not to be completely bypassed. However, even this existing content must be put through the transculturation–culture-fair–literate-fair process. Time and resources permitting, it is better to generate the content from scratch from the perspective of the target group and later synchronize it with the already-existing content in the ethnic group's native language. Such opportunities may not always exist, and the transculturation group has to move within its resources and develop the draft content.

3. **A community response panel is assembled.** The next step for the intercultural communication group is to obtain some form of response to the content that is developed from the target community. This could take the shape of a community response panel composed of lay members from the target ethnic population as well as others who are bilingually and biculturally familiar with the ethnic group's communication style and idiom—perhaps practitioners working in the target ethnic community. It may be that the available resources allow for only a few individuals to participate and not a full community response panel. In such instances the practitioners and their parent

organizations need to vary the individuals who will assist. A cross-section of lay and practitioner participants, similar to a formally constituted panel, works best. Actual numbers of participants cannot be suggested, because every situation will be different.

It is crucial that the members of this response panel or process not be anyone who participated in the actual development of the material as they will be biased one way or another toward it. The reviewers need to approach the content that has been developed independently, seeing it fresh for the first time. The task of the community response panel or individual reviewers is to then examine the material developed around two concerns: (a) does it convey information about the disorder? and (b) is it in harmony with the target ethnic group's own communicational styles and idiomatic modes of expression?

However, because either the community response panel members or the individual participants reviewing the materials that have been developed may know the original group that developed the content, there may be some hesitancy about being truly critical. However, the people conducting the review need to be told that the very best service they can give to the target ethnic community is to be both objective and truly critical. Trying to be nice to the creators of the material at this stage and letting dementing illness information errors or errors related to the cultural compatibility of the message could do harm to the ethnic community members. The reason for seeming to "step on the toes" of the intercultural communication team can also be communicated back to those involved in transculturating the original materials. Most often these matters are handled up front with the original transculturation effort group members or individuals as a part of the ground rules for the activity.

4. **This cumulative process results in a final working draft.** This draft contains the inputs of both the intercultural communication work group and the community-response panel or individual reviewers. This draft can be assembled during one or several conferences, depending on the complexity of the content. It is at this point that the content is assembled with regard to which inputs have been incorporated: (a) its overall culture fairness and (b) its literacy-level relevance.

5. **A back translation is prepared.** After completion of the above stages, a back translation into English is made of the final working draft material in the ethnic group's native language. This back translation tests the integrity of the originally intended message from another angle, namely, to determine if the information on the dementing condition being discussed has been maintained.

6. **Reconciliation of the working draft and the back translation takes place.** Discrepancies encountered between the final working draft and the back translation into English are then ironed out. A final version of the proposed content in the target group's idiom is prepared.

7. **The final document is prepared.** This last, fully transculturated, version is

then put into production and disseminated to the target ethnic group according to plan.

It is true that the overall process may appear quite detailed. However, once intercultural communication groups are formed and experience is gained, the task moves relatively smoothly. Sufficient time needs to be allotted to work through the different steps. The task may be more difficult if the content will be used for research purposes, for example, for cognitive or other types of assessment measures. In such a case the intercultural communication team needs to be certain that the items that are translated preserve the psychometric properties of the original. The effort will be less difficult for informational type communications.

The mainstream culture public at large, or even professionals and providers, may not realize how much care and attention are given to formulating Alzheimer's disease and related disorders messages in English. There are often many fine distinctions that have to be drawn so as to neither overwhelm nor confuse the audiences reading or viewing the dementing illness message. Many stereotypes about late-onset dementia still abound in the public arena. The preparation and dissemination of accurate messages about dementing illness to ethnically and linguistically diverse audiences demand equal care and attention.

A Word About Translation

The usual term used for communicating messages and information across cultures is *translation*. Say, for example, that a news story such as a new finding related to dementing illness appears in the U.S. English-language media. It is picked up from the wire services by different ethnic group media, who communicated to their audience via the audience's native language. This process can be experienced frequently by bilingual/bicultural professionals and providers in many large population centers where there are ethnically diverse media. However, if the bicultural practitioner pays close attention to the message, dementing illness focused or not, subtle changes are evident in wording and juxtaposition of ideas between the English and the other-language message. In many instances, what has happened is that the communication has been not just translated but rather transculturated, that is, the information has not been communicated literally but has been shaped so that the original intended content of the message or information is communicated to the ethnically diverse audience in the way the audience is accustomed to hearing the message.

A close observation of this process indicates that the media from other cultural groups would appear to maintain bilingual/bicultural experts on hand to make sure that the information received is presented in a culturally attuned format. The transculturation process can also be experienced at conferences where members of different language groups are in attendance. Often there are simultaneous translation services available. However, if bilingual/bicultural professionals or providers wish to verify the fact that the content is actually being transculturated rather than literally translated, they need to pay attention to the content of both languages. Individuals who are in simultaneous translator roles would seem to actually be expert transculturators who can think and communicate in the cultural contexts of both the language they are hearing and the language they are speaking.

The intercultural communication team will not always have the pressure for "instant" transculturation assistance; however, such demands can come up in many clinical situations in which the practitioner may need be sure that key information being provided in English is being understood by the linguistically diverse client group members. For example, the dementia-affected elder may be suddenly hospitalized. The staff at the hospital may ask for clarification from the family members about their wishes relative to resuscitation procedures. The ethnic group family members may in turn be quite confused by the terminology and explanations being provided in English. An outside dementia-capable practitioner who works with the ethnically diverse family members may be called in to provide on-the-spot information-transculturation assistance. As either the bilingual/bicultural professional or provider or the organization's intercultural communication team gains experience in these and other circumstances, their ability to generate culture- and literate-fair content will run progressively more smoothly.

The important point to keep in mind is that a dementing-illness message that is judged to be grammatically good or correct but that is devoid of a direct link with the target ethnic group's colloquial language and ongoing communicational style preferences may be no message at all.

A MODIFIED, PRAGMATIC APPROACH
TO THE TRANSCULTURATION PROCESS

It must be noted that what works for one linguistic group may not be automatically applicable to all others. Therefore, the suggestion is to tailor the transculturation process itself to the communication style and expectation of the target ethnic group's language. Practitioners can apply the approach that works best for their circumstances. The issue is to accomplish the effective transculturation of needed information rather than to get stuck in the process.

For example, not every practitioner will be able to assemble an intercultural work group to meet every demand for the development of culturally and linguistically compatible information. Even if the practitioners are fully bilingual or bicultural, their training and expertise may not reside in the arena of media and formal communications. Moreover, should the practitioners have such expertise, it may be difficult for them to individually go through the full transculturation process on short notice. However, there is still a way in which practitioners at this direct-service level can apply the principles outlined and be assured that the more formal messages they are relaying to the ethnically diverse families conform to the spirit of the transculturating communication process.

The fact that professionals and providers have incorporated cultural mapping/intercultural engagement techniques into their practices indicates that they are already functional transculturators of complex dementia-focused messages at the interactional level of contact. Therefore, despite the fact that they may not be experts relative to developing dementia-focused brochures, pamphlets, or other content for the media, they still can relate to the target audience by applying the approach underlying the transculturation of information for the target ethnic client group. Transculturation seeks only to make materials understood in a culture-fair way, and the practitioner may already be involved in some aspect of the effort through direct verbal exchanges with ethnically diverse client families. Since the issues are complex, a pragmatic review of a modified transculturation process is in order.

Phase 1: Starting the Transculturation

First, professional and providers, as well as the dementia-care organization, need to assemble and prioritize the intended communications that need to be transmitted to the ethnically diverse client group. In so proceeding the practitioner and the organization can proceed as follows.

1. The dementia-related content that is to be communicated in the ethnic group's language is identified.
2. A check is made to see if any of the content might not already be available in the target ethnic group's preferred language. This existing material can be used as a starting point. The professional or provider may not be able to conduct a full back translation; however, selective back translations of specific items with the existing material can reveal if it is already in a culture-fair and literate-relevant format.
3. It might be of benefit for the practitioner to see if there are materials in related health fields in the target ethnic group's preferred language. This content might have application to the dementing illness concerns. The Alzheimer's disease–dementing illness field is not the only one that speaks to issues of home safety, caregiver stress and health matters, and legal and financial planning. As in Step 2, a spot check can be made of the transculturated strength of the materials. If they pass, they might be adapted for use by the target ethnic client families.
4. At this phase of the modified transculturation process, the practitioner can reach out to key people from the target ethnic group who know how to communicate with its members. These people do not have to be expert translators; rather, what is important is to look at their bilingual/bicultural communication skills relative to the language group being accessed. The strong emphasis here is on locating bicultural communicators or brokers. There are many people who may be bilingual but who may not really know or culturally appreciate the help-seeking and help-accepting customs or normative expectations of the target ethnic group. Wherever possible, assistance from these individuals can be sought.

Phase 2: Transculturating Messages

Given that the practitioner has gone through the preceding steps as appropriate to the needs of the situation, the modified transculturation process can be fully implemented.

5. The communications/messages targeting the ethnically diverse family or larger group members are prepared.

6. The new dementia-related materials that have developed are shown to and/or discussed with the ethnic community respondents outlined in Step 4 above. The feedback from these people is incorporated into the new message prepared at this time. If already-translated dementia-pertinent content is being reviewed, or if already-translated content from allied fields will be used, judgments must be made at this time as to their linguistic and literacy relevance for the target ethnic group. If the proposed content has problems, the suggestion is not to use it, or to use only those portions that appear to communicate well to the target group.

7. With these inputs in place, the material can be seen as ready for production or distribution.

Additional Working Hints

There are other practical considerations that can make the seeming burden of transculturating messages somewhat easier.

8. The practitioner or the parent organization can keep costs down. One need not spend extravagantly to prepare a good intercultural communication document.

9. In many intercultural communication situations it is best to approach the material from a more visual standpoint. Wherever possible, the practitioner and the organization need to cut down on the use of words and technical definitions except where absolutely necessary. For example, it may be important to discuss current amyloid protein research or other aspects of Alzheimer's disease, such in response to questions about genetic linkage. However, whenver possible it is better to use pictures and graphics. In preparing ethnic-specific communications and materials it is important to tie into the group's preferred images, symbols, and even color preferences. Video and audiotape content can also be used to good effect.

10. Practitioners and the organization can also make use of local television and radio talk programs that target specific ethnic/linguistic group audiences. These are often informal in nature and can be extremely effective. However, when entering this realm the professional or provider or the organizational representative must be aware that a different type of expertise is needed. The practitioner familiar with face-to-face contacts may become uncomfortable in front of a camera or microphone. Also, the professional or practitioner using radio or television as the medium for communication has to be well versed about dementing illness, particularly if the medium is a talk show format. Many different types of calls come in, and one does not have the luxury of either looking up the information or postponing a response.

DISSEMINATION PLAN

The transculturation of the dementing illness information as described is an integral part of the overall intercultural engagement process. The materials developed have an interactive intent, that is, they are meant for active use with ethnically diverse populations to improve the health and care of the dementia-affected elder and the coping capabilities of the caregiver and family/significant others involved in the situation. Therefore, to be effective the content that is transculturated into culturally relevant formats for the target ethnic group must be accompanied by a dissemination plan.

At the level of individual ethnic client interventions, the dissemination plan can be made an integral part of the overall careplan that is developed (Anrow Sciences of Mandex, Inc., 1987). In fact, the transculturated content can be used within the LEARN problem-solving format discussed in Chapter 9. In essence, the transculturated dementia-focused material is used to educate and inform the family and caregiving significant others. The practitioner also uses the material to reinforce other aspects of the overall careplan. Finally, the professional or provider uses the transculturated content to normalize the situation being encountered and to neutralize as much as possible the negative impacts of the dementing illness circumstances being encountered.

There is, however, another level of intercultural engagement for which the practitioner and the parent dementia-care organization must develop a dissemination plan. Part Three of this book centers on the more community-wide aspects of the intercultural engagement effort. The suggestion has been made that the organization and its staff have a responsibility to transfer dementia-care information and technology to various audiences, including families at large in the ethnic community, bicultural-pairs that are formed, cultural brokers who are engaged, and the infrastructure of agencies that directly serve the target ethnic community. Each of these audiences has its own gaps in dementia-care knowledge. Each can benefit from a concerted effort to make relevant information available to them in their native languages. Each of these audiences also has its own network of contacts through which the transculturated information can be further distributed. Dementia-focused content, no matter how well prepared for the target ethnic audience, is useless if it sits unused on shelves.

There is still one further aspect of information-dissemination planning. The bulk of the discussion in this segment of the narrative has concentrated on the cultural attunement of dementia-care information for specific ethnic target groups. As has been indicated at several points in the discussion, the dementia-care organization is also faced with a multicultural social environment. Requests for assistance can come from people of many different cultural and linguistic backgrounds. Preparing transculturated dementia-relevant information for every possible ethnic group and on every dementing illness topic asked for is beyond the capability of any single local organization.

There is, however, a feasible alternative. The dementia-care organization can first, through its staff, use the intercultural knowledge base development strategies outlined in Chapter 3. The organization would then proceed with the transculturation of information process with reference to the ethnic-specific targeting approach that has been selected. At the same time, parallel to this effort, the organization and its staff would begin to collect whatever dementia content can be located that is already in the languages of other ethnic groups in the service catchment but that have not yet been targeted for services. Fortunately, there are some sources that could be solicited for these materials (Alzheimer's Disease and Related Disorders Association, 1994, Sections 10–13). Admittedly, there are still many gaps in the existing dementing-illness content covering multiple ethnic groups. However, the local dementia-care organization and its staff do not always have to start from scratch with regard to the multicultural dimension of the dementia-information–dissemination plan.

STEPS IN THE "CULTURAL ATTUNEMENT" PROCESS

There are several overarching considerations that can greatly assist in providing a direction for the cultural attunement of information for linguistically and culturally diverse audiences.

1. **The practitioner and the parent organization must focus on the intended target of the information or message rather than on the need for the message to be in another language.** The need for pertinent dementia-related information in languages other than English is ongoing. The need is not to be ignored. However, the practitioner must begin the development of the linguistically relevant content while first focusing on the intended recipients of the materials. Dementia-care organizations may feel a need to promote themselves and their programs within ethnically diverse audiences. Individual professionals or providers may likewise see a need to have materials on hand in the language of the group they may be addressing. These are commendable aims; however, serious communicational problems can arise if the message or information is not appropriately attuned to a specific ethnically diverse audience. Hence, the starting point of the cultural attunement–transculturation process is to begin the total effort with the target group in mind.

2. **The practitioner and the parent organization need to think of "transculturating" rather than "translating" the message or information.** The superiority of transculturating over translating messages and information have been elaborated throughout this chapter. However, in the press of everyday work, what can often occur is that either the practitioner or the organization will fall back into the "translating" rubric. Funds may be short. Time may be running out. Capable tranculturators may be in short supply. The demands of the ethnically diverse community for appropriate content may be urgent. The practitioner and the parent dementia-care organization may be encountering these and other types of "real world" pressures at work. Whatever the case may be, the suggestion remains to be certain that what is communicated to the target ethnic community meets the criteria enunciated earlier that: (a) the message or information is cast in behavioral terms that are understood by the

target ethnic group, (b) the message or information is conceptually in synchrony with the thinking and conceptual structure of the target ethnic group, and (c) the language used must be the one colloquially used and understood by the target ethnic group.

3. **The practitioner and the parent organization need to focus on the distribution rather than the production of the message or information.** The production of content, especially in such a complex arena as dementing illness, is without a doubt a key concern as there may be hundreds, if not thousands, of dollars involved. It is vital that the practitioner and the organization consider first who will be the recipients of the information rather than what will go into its production. The many hundreds or thousands invested in the development of the content may be wasted if the materials are not appropriately targeted relative to the factors of culture and, subsequently, literacy, as discussed above.

4. **The practitioner and the parent organization need to test the content being developed all along the way.** Here the "marketing approach" known and used by many dementia-care organizations may be quite applicable to the proposed effort. In this aspect of the strategy, the information is presented in the various stages of its development to people who may either represent or reflect the proposed eventual target audience. Such an approach can provide invaluable feedback that can be put to produce an excellently attuned final product. Depending on the available time, money, and/or staff, the marketing-feedback process can be modified so that resource constraints are taken into consideration. However, practitioners and their parent organizations run considerable risks of producing culturally inappropriate materials if they work from either the top down or in isolation from the intended ethnically diverse audience and its local normative linguistic and communicational formats.

END NOTE

With diligent planning and effort the Alzheimer's disease and related disorders message can be delivered to culturally and linguistically diverse groups. As suggested, if the practitioner is conversant with the overall cultural mapping format outlined in Part One, the transculturation process related to dementia-illness information can be considered a normal part of the day-to-day intercultural exchanges between the practitioner and the ethnic client group members. In such instances the modified transculturation process as presented above can be used to good effect.

However, when the task is the preparation and delivery of formal communications publications, such as brochures and pamphlets, as well as audio and videotapes, additional considerations come into play. Here the technological demands are more extensive, and in such instances the practitioner would be better advised to become conversant with the more complete format for transculturating messages as summarized earlier in the chapter. In this more formal communication arena practitioners need to augment their cultural mapping/intercultural engagement skills with the techniques of preparing and disseminating messages though various media. There are a number of communication resources to which one can turn relative to preparing messages for specific ethnically and linguistically diverse groups. For example, in the U.S. print media arena alone, there are several hundred ethnic-group–focused newspapers in some 40 languages, with at least 60 papers reaching the Vietnamese market alone (Sreenivasan, 1996). Many cable television outlets carry ethnically focused programming, as do the various radio stations service local areas. These resources could be asked for assistance.

Basically, the professionals or providers and the dementia-care organization have two approaches to use as they see fit. One is more or less an extension of ongoing intercultural engagement practice; the other is more demanding in that it may require the involvement of formal budget allocation and other resources. At the same time both strategies require careful attention to the conscious use of the cultural mapping/intercultural communication skills. The underlying responsibility in both approaches is that the practitioner make certain that the core content of the dementia-focused message that originates in English is transmitted in a clearly understood manner in the target ethnic group's language and at its level of understanding. Moreover, as indicated, a multitiered dissemination plan must accompany the overall cultural attunement effort.

Chapter 13

Intercultural Outreach and Networking

The cultural mapping/intercultural engagement process is put into place through the practitioner's development of community-outreach and networking skills (Alzheimer's Disease and Related Disorders Association, 1994; Aranda, 1990; Arean & Gallagher-Thompson, 1996; Banks, 1995; Brownlee, 1978; R. C. Cooley et al., 1976; Gallagher-Thompson et al., 1994; Valle, 1980b, 1988–1989; Valle & Mendoza, 1978). From an organizational standpoint, managers and directors must not only see such activity as an essential component of the overall intercultural engagement effort (Fine, 1995) but also strongly support it through resource and budget allocations. In a manner of speaking, the cultural mapping process begins and ends with outreach to the ethnocultural group. As delineated in Chapter 3, the professional or provider must reach out to gather pertinent information on the ethnocultural group being targeted for services, as well as on the multicultural social environment surrounding the dementia-care organization. From there the practitioner must begin to understand the language, customs, and beliefs of the ethnically diverse client group (Taussig & Trejo, 1992). Moving farther into the cultural mapping/intercultural engagement process, outreach and networking can be seen as an integral part of the dementia-care organization's efforts to maintain an ongoing presence in the target ethnic community as well as the multicultural environment as a whole. The organization's outreach and networking efforts can also be noted in terms of its engagement in transfer of dementia-care capabilities to the different segments of the community. The outreach and networking of the organization, as well as of the individual professional and provider, are likewise evident with regard to linking to the target ethnic community's cultural brokers.

With this said, there are some additional outreach and networking principles that require attention. This portion of the text elaborates on the more generic knowledge and skills involved in cross-cultural outreach and the networking process.

CROSS-CULTURAL OUTREACH

Cross-cultural outreach is an explicitly defined activity wherein the professionals or providers move out from their organizational home bases to engage ethnically diverse populations in their indigenous community settings. Cross-cultural outreach can use all of the standard tools of communication, including the phone, written messages, and person-to-person contact (Anrow Sciences of Mandex, Inc., 1987; Brownlee, 1978). All of the previously discussed intercultural engagement/cultural mapping skills and principles are likewise brought to bear on the outreach activity. For example, if the organization lacks the appropriate bilingual/bicultural skills, or if the individual practitioner is not bilingual/bicultural, the expectation is that the outreach effort will proceed in the context of a bicultural-pair arrangement. In some instances, when the targets of the outreach program or undertaking are themselves bilingual, a culturally sensitive monolingual English speaker can engage in the effort. However, because so many ethnically diverse group populations have large segments of monolingual native-language speakers, the professional or provider guiding the outreach approach must consider a bilingual/bicultural backup somewhere within the process.

The professional or provider contemplating the outreach effort must be ready to support the activity through a host of complementary functions; that is, the practitioner enters into the intercultural outreach enterprise in a well-planned manner (Alzheimer's Disease and Related Disorders Association, 1994; Brownlee, 1978), cognizant of reciprocity and exchange behaviors (Aranda, 1990), with an eye to timing and to the political aspects of the undertaking, as well as to the different levels of outreach activity (Brownlee, 1978, p. 95–96). The inability of the professional or provider, as well as of the parent organization, to invest the necessary time and effort and to see the outreach through its natural conclusion will lead not only to failure but also to the acquiring of a bad reputation in the target community .

Outreach Planning

First, cross-cultural outreach must be considered as a planned activity. The practitioner selects the targets of the outreach effort. Although there is always a beginning point at which one goes out fresh to the community setting, perhaps with only the name of a contact person, this should not mislead the professional or provider into neglecting to have clear objectives for the contacts being made as well as an overall plan of action. The contact person and the ethnic group members being addressed can be expected to be as busy as the practitioner. Therefore, the professionals or providers conducting the outreach need to have: (a) a clear notion of why they are making the contact, (b) a definite idea what they have to offer to those with whom the contact is being made, (c) given thought about what will be the expected outcome of the contact or session that will take place, and (d) the flexibility to handle whatever contingencies may emerge. For example, the practitioner may be going to a well-planned outreach contact session to explain the Alzheimer's disease program to an agency serving the target ethnic community. The planned discussion may turn in other directions relatively quickly.

> Case 13.1a. The bilingual/bicultural practitioner, new to the job, had arranged to go out to a senior center that served many Latino elderly. The visit had been arranged some time in advance. The practitioner was well received, and the outreach plans were being discussed. Well into the meeting, the community center director turned and asked directly: "Why did your organization pull out of the community last year without telling us anything?" The practitioner was surprised at the directness of the question but was not completely unprepared. He had done some background work and realized that a sudden change in staffing had caused the breakdown in communications. The purpose of his outreach was to repair the relationship. He recognized now that much additional relationship-proving work was needed to establish his own credibility and reestablish the relational reputation of his agency.

Outreach contacts often go quite smoothly; however, there are times when problems arise. Unless the professional or provider is prepared when difficulties come up, the outreach visit can falter, and the unprepared practitioner can leave the impression of someone who either lacks the skill or understanding to engage the target ethnic community.

Reciprocity and Exchange

Professionals or providers cannot always offer direct service "goods" to fellow practitioners and community people being contacted within the outreach effort. However, the fact that they bring dementia-related expertise may have relevance to the infrastructure of agencies and personnel serving the target ethnically diverse community. Dementia expertise itself can be considered a real commodity that the practitioner and parent organization bring to the community being targeted for the outreach undertaking.

Regardless of whether a direct, hands-on intervention is being provided or an information and referral service is being offered, the practitioner must be clear as to what type of service will actually be offered and equally explicit about its limitations. Sometimes the eagerness to please in the outreach contact taking place may override normal cautions about what the professional or provider, and/or the parent organization, can really do. The practitioners must remain cautious against promising what cannot be delivered. They must also remain alert to the fact that outreach contacts are not just visits. The parties involved in the outreach interactions are seeking to make exchanges that may enhance the scope of their respective programs or services, regardless whether these are externally funded or indigenously provided programs. The exchanges revolve around any manner of resources that can be put to use. Such resources can range from the new information that the parties bring to each other, the different skills that the parties in the outreach contact can share, or the actual provision of dementia-care services for specific ethnically diverse clients.

> Case 13.1b. The Latino practitioner faced the senior-center director's question head on. He indicated that he was sorry for the apparent break off of contact in the past by his parent dementia-care program. He indicated that as a newly hired person he brought a fresh professional attitude and that his parents had raised him to follow through with his responsibilities and that his professionalism would not let him do less. He indicated that realistically he could not promise to remain for the indefinite future, but he gave his word that, should the situation change, the director would be informed immediately.

In a world of broken commitments it would appear on the surface that the practitioner had overstated what he could or would do. After all, he could not assure his long-term employment at his parent organization, any more than any other person could. Moreover, the practitioner was new and had no track record to speak of in the community. However, it must be remembered that this was also an intercultural outreach exchange. Both parties involved were of Latino heritage. The senior center director knew that the practitioner would not mention his family upbringing in the context of the discussion if he had not meant to convey a commonly shared value about personal commitment. In many cultures that share a family–collectivist outlook, to bring one's parents and their honor into the exchange strikes a responsive chord. This does not mean that all the prior concerns are automatically obviated or that the past experience of the senior center director with the practitioner's parent organization is forgotten. This would be a naive expectation. However, the first steps in what was outlined in Chapter 5 about the initiating of culturally harmonious overtures of trust and rapport were taken, and the senior center director determined to extend the practitioner an invitation.

> Case 13.1c. After the above exchange, the senior center director indicated that he had another appointment, but he agreed to a number of specific times when the practitioner could come to talk to the center's regular membership about Alzheimer's disease and to meet with families who appeared to have an elder with memory problems. Both parted amicably.

At this point the practitioner recognized that the rupture in the relationship between his parent organization and the community setting had been repaired and that he had succeeded in establishing an initial working rapport with the center's director.

Timing, Investment of Effort, and Anxieties

In contemplating the outreach effort or program the professional or provider must make a series of determinations related to: (a) the appropriate timing of the proposed effort, (b) the amount of effort to be expended in the activity, and (c) what to do when there is a considerable lag between the initiation of the outreach effort and the expected outcome of reaching an ethnically diverse clientele. As noted, even the more experienced practitioners can experience such delays.

It can happen that neither the practitioner nor the parent agency can fully control the timing of the proposed effort. For example, the funds for the outreach program may have just been granted or, conversely, they may be delayed. In such instances, the outreach activity must be initiated, even if a different timetable is preferred, or the outreach work must be delayed past what may be considered the optimum startup time. Regardless, however, of such overarching considerations, professionals and providers do have control over both the *sequencing* of the outreach effort and the level of *input* or *investment* to be made. An example, though not directly related to dementing illness, may nonetheless help to illustrate the points being made.

Case 13.2. The Latino depression-intervention project, which had assembled and randomized 600+ middle-age Latina volunteer participants, was ready to go into the field. The project was going to use a cognitive–behavioral strategy with small groups, to be led by indigenous cultural brokers, that would meet at different locations in *barrios* (neighborhoods) where the participants lived. Suddenly the news broke that a terrible shooting had occurred in one of the key *barrios,* where at least one third of the potential participants lived. Adults and children had been injured, and some had been killed. The community was traumatized.

The Latino directors of the project found themselves under intense pressure. This was the largest study of its kind at the time. They had already used 1 year of the 3 allotted for the study to gather the participants, and the funding agency was anxious for the project get into the field.

An alternative plan was proposed that would get the small groups started in the *barrios* that had not been directly affected by the incident and then wait 6 months to start the groups in the affected *barrio.* Part of the research group argued that this step would compromise the project because word-of-mouth from the early participants would get out and affect the results of last groups to enter. The Latino project directors were aware of the research implications but decided on the alternative to give the community residents of the affected *barrio* a 6-month grieving and adjustment period.

It may be that dementia-care service personnel will not experience circumstances exactly similar to those described in Case 13.2; however, the issue at hand is that practitioners must recognize that community events will affect outreach activity. The timing, sequencing, and level of input relative to the overall outreach effort are all important considerations. Although one cannot always control the timing, the professional or provider, as well as parent organization, can affect the sequencing of the outreach activity and the extent of the effort expended.

Generally speaking, dementia-care agencies and their staff have considerable investment in the outreach effort, even in the context of a limited outreach program. To the organization, outreach represents a definite portion of budget expenditure with regard to personnel and other resources allocated to the undertaking. To the practitioner, the outreach activity might represent an investment of several months, or even longer periods, of work invested in the task. It is for these reasons that often much is expected, as well as at stake, from the outreach enterprise. However, because there can be delays between the initial investment of effort and the first positive outcomes—either in the form of invitations to the practitioner to join the target ethnic group community networks or in the context of drawing clientele from the target ethnic community—anxieties and second thoughts can enter the picture. The case just described can serve as an example, as can Case 5.2, which described delays in obtaining approval from the American Indian community, along with Case 11.4, in which the first round of outreach to the African American community floundered. As with any form of intergroup communication and interaction, "noise," delays, and stoppages can enter into the situation. The professional or provider should not become despondent; rather, an attitude of perseverance and prior acceptance by the practitioner about the uneven pace of community processes becomes a vital skill to retain in seeing the outreach activity to a fruitful outcome.

"political" Aspects of Outreach

The professional or provider cannot naively assume that the outreach effort is solely a process of meeting other practitioners and representatives of the target ethnic community to exchange information. The lowercase "p" in *political* in the title above is deliberate. Outreach activity has a political dimension (Brownlee, 1978), although not in the sense of the politics that accompanies the elective process. For example, the practitioner must at times meet with the leaders of a community, that is, with the people identified in Chapter 11 (Box 11.2) as coming from the "power networks." The practitioner's parent dementia-care organization may, objectively speaking, have a low level of influence. The practitioner may be even lower on the scale of relative power or influence. Still, the fact that the organization has some resources in the form of the knowledge it has or the services it can offer is a form of power; that is, the organization has "goods" to provide. Moreover, the outreach professional or provider brings personal competencies to the outreach engagement process. It is in this context of goods and resources that outreach can be considered political.

Practitioners and their parent dementia-care organizations may not be attracted to this aspect of outreach. What can mitigate the power and influence concerns is the stressing of the intercultural reciprocity and rapport aspects of the exchanges that take place. A focus on service objectives as opposed to resource-control aims can likewise assist in keeping the outreach effort on its original intercultural track. In this manner, the community contacts will come to recognize that the professional's and provider's orientations remain focused on dementia care. Not all practitioners are either attracted to what has been noted here as the political side of outreach or have the skills to function at this level. In such instances the parent organization may need to look to other staff resources to provide the necessary level of community engagement required to maintain a fruitful outreach effort.

Different Levels of Outreach

Outreach activity can proceed at different levels in either a separate or concurrent manner. For example, the outreach can take the form of direct contacts with: (a) dementia-affected elders and their caregiving family members/significant others, (b) indigenous community groups and associations, (c) the community's cultural brokers, and (d) professional and provider peers who are equally active in the target community. Each of these facets of outreach has special considerations that need to be examined.

For example, if the focus of the outreach effort is on client contact and recruitment, the potential political aspects of the outreach activity may not even appear, and the cultural mapping/cultural engagement considerations discussed throughout Parts One and Two would predominate. The same perspective would apply if the practitioner were reaching out to local community groups, such as senior citizens or parents, or self-help associations. In such instances the professional's or provider's emphasis would remain on contacting members of the target ethnocultural group to potentially attract and serve clients.

If, however, the practitioner were to engage the civic and/or business organizations in the target ethnic community, the focus might shift to take in the broader spectrum of outreach considerations being discussed. In many ethnically diverse communities there are often counterparts to, or chapters of, mainstream civic associations, such as Lions, Rotarians, chambers of commerce, and a host of other groups. In such cases the practitioners would be coming closer to contacting the ethnocultural community's leaders as representatives of their parent organizations, or as experts in the area of dementing illness. Here the "influence" factor may be operating in the context that the professional or provider may be seeking to influence the leadership to put dementing illness higher on the priority list of the audiences' list of interests and concerns.

When the outreach is focused on the ethnocultural group's cultural brokers, the outreach may once again shift in emphasis. As outlined in Chapter 11, these individuals are service focused; hence the professional or provider must be prepared to highlight the manner in which the ongoing contact would be of benefit to the target ethnic community and the families with which they may be in direct contact. The "influence" factor here is that the professional or provider has something to offer the community, and the association between the practitioner and the cultural broker can bring needed resources to bear on community needs.

Finally, if the outreach is directed to practitioner peers in the community who are staffing or directing the infrastructure of agencies and organizations serving the target ethnic community, the outreach emphasis would shift once again. Here the professionals or providers can be seen as intraorganizational in nature, that is, they have to understand the manner in which different organizations operate in the same "shared" service environment without necessarily "sharing" the same goals. Moreover, even though practitioners may be coming in the context of representing themselves, they are often seen as representatives of their parent organizations with all of the organization's strengths, weaknesses, and historical presence in the community. The practitioner in Case 13a, b, and c found himself walking the fine line between presentation of self and the past negative presence of his parent organization in the target ethnocultural community.

Basically, the professional or provider engaged in outreach must be alert to all of the different facets of the community and the varied levels at which outreach activity operates. It is not that the ethnic group practitioner peers and community groups are unresponsive or uncaring about the needs of families, and specifically those of dementia-affected people; rather, the issue is that practitioners must be ready to address service system and community-wide concerns alongside client issues.

Bicultural-Pair and Outreach

Outreach by the bicultural-pair requires special considerations. The monocultural English-speaking member of the bicultural-pair will have the primary expertise related to knowledge of dementing illness and the goals of the parent organization. The monocultural practitioner may even professionally outrank the bicultural team member. However, when directly engaging the community contacts the monocultural team member must accept the cultural guidance of the bicultural member of the effort. After all, the rationale for forming the bicultural-pair in the first place was to merge the dementia expertise with the cultural expertise. The expectation is that the style of the intercultural outreach engagement and the procedures by which the bicultural-pair will guide itself will be worked out well in advance of the actual moment of contact.

Case 4.3 highlights some of the issues in terms of how a monocultural dementia-capable practitioner and a bilingual/bicultural Navajo cultural broker worked out the separate but complementary roles. Both the individual professional or provider, and the field of dementia-care as a whole, can learn much about intercultural exchanges from the capabilities of the indigenous members of the bicultural-pair. At the same time, the bicultural-pair's professional interaction is not just one-sided. There is much that the bicultural member of the team can learn about the mainstream culture. Certainly, almost by definition, it can be said that this team member has acquired the knowledge and skill to cross two cultures. However, this may be a somewhat simplified view. As indicated at the onset, in the introduction to Part One, mainstream culture is in itself quite diverse with respect to regional and generational cultural defenses. Therefore, there is much of a cultural nature, beyond dementia-care knowledge and skills, that can be exchanged with the ethnically diverse member of the bicultural-pair. This part of the exchange of capabilities can form a part of the culturally reciprocal aspects of the bicultural-pair relationship with reference to outreach activity or any other aspect of joint dementia-care intervention. Maintaining a bidirectional cultural learning emphasis can also serve to strengthen the overall contributions that the team can make.

Multicultural Outreach

Most of the emphasis up to this point has been placed on ethnic-specific outreach. Nevertheless, multicultural outreach activity also needs to be considered (Valle, 1980b; 1981). This impetus can come from an ethnically diverse community where several ethnically diverse groups may come forward to ask for information about and assistance with dementing illness. The impetus for multicultural outreach can come also from the dementia-care organization itself, whose directors and managers have determined to prioritize engagement with several cultures. Regardless of the direction from which the multicultural outreach activity begins, the rule of thumb is to expand the bicultural-team effort to be able to cover the mix of ethnically diverse target audiences. Several bicultural-pair arrangements can be formed, some more temporary, some more permanent, as the need may be. As has already been indicated, individuals who are bicultural at times have the orientations and skills to cross more than two cultures. By being able to bridge once from their own to another culture, the potential is there to bridge to other cultures also. The central difficulty that may arise, however, is that there is a need to communicate to all of the ethnically diverse groups in their own native languages. Here, just the willingness to relate across cultures may not be enough. In this case the bicultural-pair must be able to communicate in each ethnic group's native idiom especially where monolingual ethnically diverse elderly and caregivers are concerned.

Organization's Commitment to Outreach

As discussed in Chapter 10, the assumption made is that the dementia-care organization with which the bilingual/bicultural professional or provider or bicultural-pair is affiliated supports the effort. Obviously, such a generalization will not hold up in many situations. In any number of instances, the outreach will be initiated and maintained by a small component of the organization. In others, the outreach may be sustained primarily by an individual professional or provider who sees the community needs and accepts the responsibilities involved.

However, it is only when the outreach has the full support of the parent dementia-care organization that the effort moves ahead strongly. When the support for the outreach comes only from the fringe of the organization, or from activity of an individual practitioner, certain safeguards must be put into place. First, as indicated earlier, the practitioner must be cautious about committing to what cannot be delivered. When great need is encountered, it is difficult to resist overextending the outreach effort and promising more than can be given in the interest of offering assistance. Nonetheless, practitioners must stay within the bounds of what can actually be provided, whether this is only dementia-care information or limited dementia-care assistance. Second, if one of the intended outcomes of the outreach is to bring the ethnically diverse family to the parent organization, the practitioner needs to either prepare the parent dementia-care organization for the arrival of the ethnically diverse family, accompany the family to the setting, or do both. Case 10.1a and 10.1b illustrates what can happen when unintended events interfere with the ability of the single bilingual/bicultural staff member to be present when the family members arrive. A way to obviate the difficulties has already been outlined with regard to the careful planning activity that needs to accompany the outreach effort.

INTERCULTURAL NETWORKING

Intercultural networking is a natural outcome of outreach. Networking is based on the premise that the target community is "naturally" organized (Fellin, 1995; Suttles,

1972; Warren, 1955) and has its own "folkways" (Kinneman, 1947), although the folkways and organization may not be centered around dementing illness. Networking reaches back to what Lewin (1936) highlighted as "topological space," where the person and others come into contact with each other within the social environment. Networking involves the professional's or provider's engagement with the many different layers of interactive systems present in the community (Biegel, Shore, & Gordon, 1982; Naparastek, Biegel, & Spiro, 1982; Rivera & Erlich, 1992; Warren, 1955, 1973; Yancy Martin & O'Connor, 1989). It carries with it the notion of the establishment of alliances with the many actors in the interorganizational environment and of "coalition building" (Netting, Kettner, & McMurtry, 1993; Tropman, Erlich, & Rothman, 1995). By networking, the practitioner is extending the organization's commitment to the community (Alzheimer's Disease and Related Disorder Association, 1994).

Networking also presupposes that all of the different aspects just discussed with regard to outreach are likewise being observed. This means that the professional or practitioner engaged in networking (a) follows through with planning the networking involvement, (b) remains alert to the intercultural engagement reciprocity and exchange dynamics expressed through the sharing of expertise and services, (c) remains equally alert to the timing of the network activity as well as the overall investment of time and energy required, (d) is cognizant of the political aspects of the networking processes, and (e) is prepared to engage in different levels of networking activity. If the outreach effort has been conducted well, the networking can get underway. If some aspects of the outreach remain unresolved, the ability of the professional or provider to fully follow through with the networking phase may be impaired.

On the positive side, a well-conducted outreach campaign brings with it active networking membership. However, network memberships also bring additional task considerations for the practitioner, as there usually are many different networks and activities going on within any given community. To this end, the professionals and providers need to carefully consider their involvements and commitments to the different networks they engage.

Case 13.3a. The bicultural practitioner from the dementia-care clinic affiliated with a local teaching hospital had been active for some time in outreach to the African American community. She had been bringing the dementia-care message to various groups and centers in the area. On the same day, the senior adult day health programs coalition chair, and the regional provider's council, called and invited her to be a member of their groups. She found herself in a quandary, because she was already assigned to other ongoing community-liaison responsibilities. She felt that attending at least one of the new networks would be helpful, as both were specifically focused on the community where she was conducting her outreach. As a nurse, she favored the adult day program's coalition because of the affinity to her profession; however, the provider's council really dealt more directly with her area of responsibility. Perhaps because she and her supervisor attended the senior adult day health coalition together she could ask for a release of responsibilities to one group and take on the region provider's council responsibility.

Crisscross Networking

As practitioners enter the network process they will find not only a proliferation of networks but also interlocking memberships by many of the same practitioners; for example, the member of one council or coalition will be the chairperson or officer of another network organization. Many members of one council or coalition will see each other one day early in the month at one meeting and perhaps at another later the next week. This type of redundancy is not necessarily negative; rather, the ongoing contacts allow the network members to exchange information on an ongoing basis.

Case 13.3b. The bicultural practitioner had been working on an especially difficult case. Mrs. Anderson, a 73-year-old African American woman, had been living alone. A fall brought her to the community hospital. There the staff had called the hospital's affiliated outpatient dementia-care clinic for an evaluative consultation as a dementing disorder was suspected. Through the eventual workup, Mrs. Anderson was diagnosed as having probable Alzheimer's disease in the early moderate stage. The practitioner was working with the hospital discharge planner to find a suitable placement for the patient, as no family members could be located. The intake staff member of an Alzheimer's special-care unit that had two open Medicaid beds. The special care unit intake worker and the bicultural practitioner had been leaving messages for each other for several days. They finally met at the provider's council session and were able to expedite Mrs. Anderson's placement when she would be released from the hospital.

Meetings such as those described immediately above can serve many networking purposes, including resolution of case management issues.

Role Consistency in Networking

Another important aspect of networking is the fact that the participants become well-known to each other. Through networking one often gets to know one's referral sources on a firsthand basis. This can be of considerable benefit to the professional or provider, especially when putting complex careplans together. For example, an additional complexity turned up with regard to Mrs. Anderson that needed quick attention

Case 13.3c. Mrs. Anderson's neighbors had said that one of the other residents in the apartment building where she lived assisted Mrs. Anderson in cashing her checks and in keeping current with paying bills and daily needs purchases. No one could locate the neighbor or the records, and an adult protective-services worker became involved. The practitioner and the adult protective-services worker arranged to meet at the provider's council, where all the concerns were resolved. Mrs. Anderson's helper had been visiting an out-of-state daughter for 3 weeks and knew nothing of the events leading up to Mrs. Anderson's hospitalization or the subsequent events leading to the money concerns. She was only too glad now that her friend would get good care.

There is another advantage to the crisscrossing and interlocking community networks. These linkages allow the professional and provider to demonstrate the consistency of their role performance in a relatively short time. The dementia-care practitioners not only observe other network members, but they also find themselves likewise in the spotlight. Networks have a form of a reputational multiplier effect. The dementia-care practitioner who is aware of this aspect of networking dynamics can communicate not only a consistency of purpose but also necessary knowledge about dementing illness and supportive interventions. This element of networking is especially important to professionals who are new to the area, such as those described in Case 13.1a, 13.1b, and 13.1c. The same features can be found in Case 7.3, in which a new bilingual/bicultural Japanese American practitioner joined the area's Alzheimer's network, as well as in those cases involving links to the ethnic group's cultural brokers, such as Case 11.2, with regard to the Haitian community, in Case 11.3, with the Latino community, and in Case 11.4, with reference to the African American group.

Networking and Organizational Role Conflicts

There is an additional important consideration regarding networking and the parent dementia-care organization. At times there may be several different practitioners assigned networking responsibilities. This situation occurs most commonly if the organization is especially large, but it can happen in moderately sized or small dementia-care organizations where there is a need to engage the community networks on behalf of multiple clients. The circumstance can likewise come up when staff from different personnel levels in the organization begin to engage the same community networks. For example, the managers may be networking at one level and the direct-service professionals or providers at another.

In all of these different circumstances, the practitioners from the same parent organization who are similarly engaged in the networking activity must communicate the same overall message. They can relate to their particular organizational roles and responsibilities, as well as to their professional or provider specialties and training. However, the organizational message with regard to dementia care, and especially with respect to the ethnically diverse groups whose members are now part of the organization's client population, must be consistent. This means that the different personnel have to find ways to communicate and keep each other abreast of important items that occur. For example, in the case of Mrs. Anderson (Case 13.3a, b, and c), events moved relatively swiftly, the practitioner would have needed to inform her supervisor, who was networking in the same community setting of what was transpiring. Consistency of performance in the networking environment is assessed in terms not only of the individual practitioner's track record, but also of the records of all the other members of the same organization who may be active in the same community or working on the same tasks.

Case 13.4. The dementia-care organization had assigned several personnel to work on different aspects of the community work in preparation for National Alzheimer's month. The theme this year was "the multicultural face of Alzheimer's." In addition, several bilingual/bicultural members of the organization's governing board volunteered to take active roles and began meeting with the respective ethnic groups with which they were affiliated. The executive director was quite pleased that so many parts of the agency were involved. She was nevertheless concerned that there seemed to be little internal coordination within the organization relative to this important undertaking. She drew her evidence from the phone calls to her from community leaders seeking clarification of the different kinds of information they were receiving. She talked the matter over with the chair of the governing board. A temporary task force was created, and all the different personnel from the agency who had been assigned networking duties for the upcoming multiculturally focused Alzheimer's month events were made members. The organization's outreach coordinator was appointed as the task force chair. This change brought about a resolution of the role-and-message confusion that was affecting the overall networking effort.

As illustrated in Case 13.4, there are many positives to having an active commitment from different sectors of the organization. However, quality control is a necessary ingredient to assure consistency within the organization's overall networking activity.

Multicultural Versus Ethnic-Specific Networking

Most of the time intercultural networking is multi-ethnic in scope, that is, the members of the practitioners in the service-oriented networks may themselves be of many different ethnic backgrounds. This is very often the case even where the network itself may be targeting one or more specific ethnic groups. Moreover, these networks will most likely be multidisciplinary in nature, because often different practitioners from different specialities or disciplines find that they need to engage with peers from other fields to resolve the problems or issues on which the network is focusing.

The professional or provider, as well as the parent organization, is likewise just as likely to encounter ethnic-specific networks within the same environment. The more ethnic-specific networks will emerge especially around the search for cultural brokers and for clients from specially targeted ethnic populations. Cases 13.1a, b, and c can serve as examples of outreach where the supportive networking would need to be more ethnic specific. Case 5.2, with regard to the dementia-needs assessment among the Native American tribal councils, also could serve as an example of more ethnic-specific networking. In contrast, Cases 13.3a, 13.3b, and 13.3c, with regard to Mrs. Anderson's needs, Case 5.1, in which the dementia-care organization was focused on several ethnic groups, and Case 13.4 would all illustrate the need for multicultural networking support.

Consistent with wherever in the text the theme of multicultural versus ethnic-specific intercultural engagement has been discussed, the professional and provider, and the parent dementia-care organization must be ready to respond in both directions. The pattern of the community needs or individual family needs, or the issues that are encountered, may all dictate the practitioner's and the organization's response. Both sets of capabilities must be built into the practitioner's and organization's repertoire of skills.

Cultural–Historical Presence of Networks

In many, if not most, instances, professionals and providers will find that they are entering existing networks that have been in place for some time. It is not that new networks cannot be formed to meet emerging needs but rather that the networks for the most part will contain individuals who have been in place and in network activist roles for some time. In such instances, the approaches suggested throughout Chapter 3 with respect to formulating cultural–historical insight into a specific ethnic group or multicultural region can be modified to gather the background about the network's own historical presence. Group process of almost any sort creates a historical–contextual process of normative behaviors and expectations (Yancy Martin & O'Connor, 1989, pp. 165–168). The new person entering the group—in this case, the dementia-care practitioner—is well served by knowing this process background. For one thing, such knowledge will enable the professional or provider to understand the "cultural rules" of the network, as the network in itself becomes a "mini-culture" (Valle, 1985).

Marketing, Outreach, and Networking

The topic of marketing, and especially of marketing to ethnically diverse populations, is, in and of itself, a topic needing serious attention (Alzheimer's Disease and Related Disorders Association, 1994). Dementia-care organizations in particular, and the field of dementia care as a whole, are in need of cross-cultural marketing expertise. Not enough marketing is being done to include ethnically diverse populations in the distribution of available dementia-care products, care strategies, and programs. However, in the context of the discussion here, marketing on the one hand and outreach and networking on the other are complementary but quite different approaches to the issue of extending dementia-care resources to ethnocultural diverse groups. The suggestion, therefore, is to avoid mixing the messages. Outreach and networking as discussed in this segment of the text are not generating customers for a new product but rather are extending dementia-care services to clients with specific needs to be met. Although the organization needs to have the capabilities in both areas of effort, each type of function—outreach and networking on one hand, and marketing on the other—has its separate rationale and function. They need to be seen as complementary rather than synonymous activities.

OUTREACH AND NETWORKING PRINCIPLES: A BRIEF SUMMARY

1. **The practitioner needs to consider the intended outcomes at the start of the outreach and networking activity.** Prior planning and the ongoing examination of the directions in which the outreach and networking activity is proceeding are the order of the day, so to speak, for the professional or provider and the organization. The eventual linkage of dementia-care services to ethnically diverse populations in need requires a carefully planned as well as a flexible approach to the work that is undertaken.

2. **Both outreach and networking are conducted in complex social environments. The dementia-care practitioner needs to remain on track with respect to the original intercultural engagement mission that is undertaken.** Outreach and networking relationships, as well as the communicational processes involved, move quickly. The practitioner has to be able to handle the changes that arise from all of the different interactions that take place. This is best done if the original intercultural engagement objectives are constantly kept in mind.

3. **It will be of benefit to the practitioner to apply the cultural mapping rules and principles outlined earlier in the discussion to the outreach and networking enterprise.** Outreach and networking take place in cultural environments, whether these be the ethnocultural groups being targeted for with the activity or the people who come together in the community-service networks. The cultural mapping strategies can be applied in either area.

4. **Outreach and networking are not private undertakings; both take place in very public contexts.** The professional or practitioner, and the parent organization, plays very public roles in both outreach and networking. What is said and done in an individual outreach contact or a networking meeting is disseminated throughout the network. The purpose of the networks is to do just that—namely, to get pertinent information out to the members. The practitioner needs to enter this communicational environment consciously alert to this fact. Positive and negative messages move out quickly.

END NOTE

Intercultural outreach and networking within the target ethnically diverse community are integral and ongoing components of the professionals' and providers' roles in seeking to engage ethnically diverse populations (Valle, 1988–1989). In doing so the practitioner and the parent dementia-care organization communicate a willingness to extend dementia services to potentially underserved populations. The provider or practitioner also indicates an implicit understanding of the ground rules of working effectively in the target community. Although the topics of outreach and networking have been discussed somewhat separately, they are really two sides of the same coin. What is crucial for the practitioner and the parent dementia-care organization is to also see that outreach and networking are a natural extension of the cultural mapping/ intercultural engagement process.

Chapter 14

Highlighting Issues and Looking Ahead

INTERCULTURAL ENGAGEMENT: SELF-MONITORING OVERVIEW

From time to time the professional or provider, as well as the parent dementia-care organization, will need to undertake an overview of the status of the intercultural effort that is being implemented. Such an exercise can be helpful in identifying the strong points of the effort along with pinpointing areas that may require concerted attention. The *Intercultural Engagement Performance Monitoring Log,* delineated in Box 14.1, can be quite useful for this purpose. The issue is not that the log itself should be used slavishly, but rather that the practitioner and the parent organization are monitoring the direction and outcomes of the cross-cultural engagement activity that has been undertaken.

It is recognized that the dementia-care service-related demands can become intense. It may, therefore, be easy to lose sight of the broader picture of all of the different factors involved in intercultural engagement with ethnically diverse populations. To this end the log (Box 14.1) is provided. Because it is a summarized list only, practitioners are encouraged to modify it to suit the circumstances of their interventive situations. The log covers four major areas: (1) the documentation of the practitioner's and/or the parent dementia-care organization's cross-cultural awareness quotient and overall intercultural engagement capabilities; (2) the delineation of the planned support for the intercultural engagement effort to be provided by the parent dementia-care organization; (3) the identification of the practitioner's and parent

1. CROSS-CULTURAL CAPABILITIES AND AWARENESS	THE SPECIFIC DOMAIN IS: IN PLACE/GAPS EXIST/MISSING
1.1 The target ethnocultural community's perceptions and level of knowledge of dementing illness are identified and understood.	
1.2 The ethnocultural community's ethnocultural perceptions about needs of patients and the help-seeking and help-accepting behaviors of caregivers and family members are also identified and understood.	
1.3 The planned approach has been tailored to local conditions and circumstances.	
1.4 An overall attempt is maintained to harmonize with the values of the target ethnic group, even if these are seen as at variance with the outreach organization's notions of what is "good" or "best."	
2. PARENT DEMENTIA-CARE ORGANIZATION PLANNED SUPPORT	
2.1 The outreach effort is embedded in the sponsoring organization's policies.	
2.2 It has the support of the governing board of the organization and its managers.	
2.3 Budget and other resources have been allocated to facilitate the effort.	
2.4 There is a long-range plan in place, accompanied by short-term operational goals.	
2.5 The outreach effort is accompanied by a monitoring and evaluation plan.	
3. OUTREACH/NETWORKING STRATEGIES	
3.1 The key local cultural brokers and bicultural-pair candidates have been identified.	
3.2 There is a mechanism for continued expansion of the cultural broker/bicultural-pair pool.	
3.3 An understanding of the different levels of cultural brokers and the various roles they play has been attained.	
3.4 Overreliance on family caregiver go-betweens/brokers is avoided.	

3. OUTREACH/NETWORKING STRATEGIES	THE SPECIFIC DOMAIN IS: IN PLACE/GAPS EXIST/MISSING
3.5 The principles of reciprocity guide the networking strategy. This includes the transfer of technology to the target ethnic community.	
4. COMPATIBLE COMMUNICATION TECHNIQUES ARE IN PLACE AND REGULARLY EMPLOYED 4.1 Information and referral materials are available in transculturated/culture-fair formats in the appropriate target ethnic group's language.	
4.2 Culturally and linguistically appropriate and dementing-illness information and referral support services are incorporated.	
4.3 An ongoing interactive communicational approach is utilized. Wherever possible, media (radio, television, print), attuned to the language and culture of the target ethnic group, are employed.	
4.4 The materials also are in literate-fair formats.	
4.5 The culture-fair/literate-fair formats are extended to the dementia-care organization's formal communications also.	

Box 14.1 Intercultural engagement performance monitoring log.

organization's outreach and networking strategies, including the engagement of cultural brokers and bicultural-pairs; and (4) the deployment of culturally compatible communication techniques. All of the other more specific aspects of the cultural mapping/intercultural engagement process have already been detailed and summarized in their appropriate chapters. In fact, the log presented here can be combined with the Cultural Mapping/Intercultural Assessment Checklist (Box 9.1) presented in Chapter 9. Together they can serve as a form of management information system (MIS) for tracking the overall cross-cultural activity that is initiated. In an MIS format both the log and the checklist can serve to track both quantitative and qualitative intercultural engagement data.

CORE PURPOSE OF CULTURAL MAPPING PROCESS

The professional or provider working in the intercultural arena must recognize that cultures wear many veils (Valle, 1990a). As one is pulled aside, another appears immediately behind it. This should not be surprising. As indicated in Chapter 2, despite their apparent inertia, cultures are constantly evolving, and so are the group members of specific ethnocultural groups. Even though there may be a tendency among many ethnically diverse group members to deeply value their group's traditions, variations on the original cultural themes will emerge, especially in the context of a quickly evolving host society such as the United States. Therefore, the practitioner has to know how to identify an ethnic group's traditional outlooks while at the same time remaining flexible to accommodate the changes that have occurred through acculturation pressures (Montalvo & Gutierrez, 1989; Paniagua, 1994; Westermeyer, 1987).

The cultural mapping strategy outlined throughout the text is designed to assist the professional or provider in handling what were earlier noted as the more "fixed" (or traditional) and the more "fluid" (or acculturating) aspects of the ethnically diverse client group members' lives. The suggested approach enables the practitioner to establish an ongoing interactive rapport with the members and to bring the dementia care provided to a successful and culturally compatible conclusion. Given the nature of dementing illness and the eventual outcome for the affected person, the intercultural engagement process is also about helping the ethnically diverse group members through their culturally relevant grieving customs (Kawaga-Singer, 1994; Pickett, 1993). Cultural mapping must therefore be understood to be about beginnings, about ongoing relational processes, and about reaching appropriate closure with ethnically diverse populations. With this noted, a few additional remarks are in order.

Disease, Illness, and Culture

Throughout the preceding discussion, professionals and providers have been urged to separate the *disease entity* that may be present in dementing conditions and the *illness response process* of the affected people and their caregiving significant others. Kleinman (1977, 1986a, 1986b) has spoken to this point with more general reference to illness, and Christensen and Jorm have addressed this (1992) with regard to the area of dementia. If the diagnosis is that of probable Alzheimer's disease, the professional or provider can be certain that physiological damage is being done to the affected person's brain, regardless of ethnicity. This damage is not reversible. The process to be encountered will be one of a gradual degenerative decline evidenced in the person's loss of short-term memory capabilities; loss of language and reasoning capacity; growing disorientation to time and place, and of eventual major impairments in basic motor functions. The affected person is thereby forced to live more and more in the distant past of the long-term memory, where many coping behaviors were first enculturated. The point of the intercultural engagement emphasis of the text, therefore, has been on providing interventive approaches that may enhance the patient's current situation by establishing *culturally compatible* behavioral and affective links between needs and service resources.

The point of the intercultural interventive emphasis of the discussion has also been on establishing these same behavioral and affective links with the ethnically diverse dementia-affected person's caregiving family members and significant others. It is here that the issues of culture and ethnicity likewise surface and will be expressed in the language and communication patterns, interaction formats, customary caregiving practices, values, beliefs, and normative expectations in regard to dementing-illness care concerns. In essence, the target ethnocultural group members will be expressing their cultural orientations in terms of their responses to the problems encountered.

The dementing condition will be present, and the reactions will vary. The *interculturally proficient practitioner* is one who is able to distinguish between the "illness" issues and the underlying "disease condition" quite naturally without a second's hesitation.

Remaining Culture Neutral

Intercultural practice does not place a value of one culture over another. Each culture, being a human invention, has its strengths and its limitations. The cultural mapping process is directed toward identifying and working with the variations that are found. In this context, the professional or provider enters the dementia-care situation looking to recognize the wide spectrum of attitudinal and behavioral responses among ethnically diverse client group members. The practitioner's assessment, therefore, is based not on determining whether cultures are "good" or "bad" but rather on how the ethnically diverse client group's coping strategies assist or impede dementia-affected people and their caregiving significant others

In this regard, the professional or provider remains *culturally neutral* with respect to placing an external value on a particular set of beliefs or customs actively used by the members of a specific ethnic group. The practitioner's perspective should be focused on how a particular set of outlooks or practices can facilitate or hinder the dementia-care circumstances of both the patient and the caregiving significant others. The expectation throughout the cultural mapping approach is that the act of linking to the client group's normally accepted ways of coping will reduce the stresses associated with dementia caregiving. A further expectation is that by recognizing and respecting the ethnically diverse client's values and outlooks, the professional or provider will be able to provide a bridge for the clients to access the resources available in the dementia-care field. The hope is to meet the dementia patient's needs and to ease the caretaking burden in a manner that uses as many of the ethnic group members' cultural strengths as possible. As noted in the earlier discussion, it is difficult for even trained practitioners to assume this perspective. *Ethnocentrism* is ever present, particularly the ethnocentrism toward one's own professional or provider culture. Remaining centered on one's own worldviews is a very powerful force for the practitioner and the layperson alike. The intercultural engagement process, with its specific cultural attunement strategies and techniques, is oriented toward neutralizing the potential intrusive impact of one's worldview into the dementia-care intervention situation. As has been noted above, even the bilingual/bicultural professional or provider must be cautious about imposing personal perspectives into the dementia-care circumstances that are encountered, even with people of one's own culture of origin.

At the same time, remaining *culture neutral* does not in any way imply that the practitioner is to remain unresponsive in situations in which culturally unique linguistic, interactional, and value orientations within ethnically diverse caregiving contexts may be inappropriately impacting care for the dementia-affected elder. Here the practitioner must move delicately and proactively to identify where cultural preferences of the ethnically diverse client group may be impeding the dementia-care situation. At the same time, the professional or provider must remain alert to a wholesale attempt to replace cultural preferences and approaches. The application of the LEARN problem-solving formation discussed in Chapter 9 can be of considerable benefit in such situations. In this context, the practitioner works closely with the ethnically diverse client group, at times modeling behaviors that are both culturally compatible to the ethnic group members and of assistance to the dementia-affected elder.

Dementing Illness, Ethics, and Culture

The discussion of ethnocentrism and the need for *values neutrality* on the part of the practitioner extends to another crucial aspect of dementing illness. This is when value and value differences, namely ethical decision-making, come into play, especially around *advance directives* and end-of-life circumstances. The problem is made more difficult because in dementing illness, the patient is usually surrounded by proxy decision-makers, whether these are family members, someone appointed by the court, or a public body. The question then becomes not just whose values or what mix of values is involved, but also to what extent the dementia-affected person's own wishes and judgments can be discerned and followed. A struggle emerges between what Kapp (1994, p. 35) calls the "values of autonomy and beneficience." Very often in the earlier stages of a dementing condition, patients can in some way make their wishes known. However, the circumstances always vary according to the course of the dementing condition within the individual (Sachs and Cassell, 1989). Therefore, the individual patient's decision-making capabilities; the benevolent interests of others, whether they are family members, providers, or court appointed surrogates; and culturally held values all come together into a thorny problem (Buchanan and Brock, 1986).

The topic is too broad to be covered in this portion of the text. Nonetheless, the literature is informative relative to ways to approach the issues of ethical decision-making and dementing illness from a cross-cultural perspective. Welsh et al. (1994) stress the need to clarify how culture and status differences between ethnically diverse clients and practitioners impact informed consent processes. Bedolla (1995) and Kawanga-Singer (1994) both urge the practitioner to keep in mind that the ethical values of one culture may not be mutually shared by other cultures or prioritized in the same manner. For example, some cultures may place priority on the principle of autonomy that is prized within the U.S. mainstream culture. Pickett (1993, p. 105) offers a series of practical suggestions centering around the notion of employing *cultural brokerage* where messages, instructions, and belief systems are exchanged between cultural groups. Draguns's (1996) principle that the practitioner must be able to distinguish what is humanly universal from what is culturally distinctive in the intercultural engagement process is especially applicable to the cross-cultural ethics arena. Case 8.1a and 8.1b are illustrative of practitioners encountering ethical values differences where such concepts have direct bearing. The cultural assessment and intervention principles and practices delineated throughout Parts One and Two of the text can likewise be extended to the ethical decision-making arena.

Dementia-Care Emphasis/Other Ethnic Group Needs

Although the overall discussion has centered on dementing illness and culturally appropriate dementia-care strategies, the professional or provider working with ethnically diverse client family groups will often be confronted with a host of other attendant needs and problems. To a large extent these circumstances are a consequence of the group members being isolated from mainstream informational and service resources. Therefore, if a culturally compatible relationship is established, with all of the attendant trappings of rapport and trust, the dementia-care professional or provider can expect requests for assistance to be made with respect to these other areas of need beyond dementing illness.

In such instances the practitioner will have to act according to the availability of time and other service-provision skills and capabilities. Wherever possible, the professional or provider is encouraged to respond to the requests made. It is here also that the problem-solving LEARN formulation presented in Chapter 9 may be put to additional practical use.

Broader Aspects of Cultural Mapping Model

The central focus of the discussion has been on implementing culturally relevant strategies within the dementia-care arena. However, it should be noted that cultural mapping techniques are applicable to many other areas of service and interaction with ethnically diverse populations. For example, the suggested individual or family client-oriented approaches for rapport and trust building are adaptable to many other facets of intergroup intercultural engagement. Similarly, the acculturation continuum formulation, a component of the overall model, can be made relevant to the ongoing interaction between the ethnic group members and the host society in regard to a variety of issues and concerns. Professionals and providers from related fields of service, and outside the sphere of dementia care, can therefore feel free to make use of or adapt the ideas as presented here. The manifestation of culturally based beliefs, attitudes, and behaviors are not restricted to the dementing-illness arena alone. Moreover, as noted at the onset of the narrative, help-seeking and help-accepting normative expectations extend to most, if not all ethnic groups and their endeavors. In this context, English-speaking Euro-Anglo mainstream ethnic group members may likewise benefit from the introduction of cultural mapping techniques into the services regularly provided to them.

Intercultural Engagement: A Different Direction

The discussion as a whole has also focused on the act of intercultural engagement coming from the bilingual/bicultural professional or provider, or the bicultural-pair, and directed to the ethnically diverse client group. The intercultural engagement strategy of giving attention to the ethnic client group's traditional, culture-of-origin outlooks have been outlined in detail. There is, however, a very different need that is manifesting itself throughout the dementia-care field as a whole and that is most often being noticed in residential or skilled-nursing facilities. As of this writing, many of the clienteles of these facilities come primarily from mainstream U.S., English-speaking Anglo-ethnic host society cultural backgrounds. On the other hand, the direct-care staff, particularly at the aide level, may come from quite ethnically diverse backgrounds. Communicational and intercultural behavioral misunderstandings are common. Neither side clearly understands the other and, despite good intentions, if dementing illness is present, the misunderstandings can become quite pronounced and persistent, escalating into personnel problems as well as into ongoing resident/client–staff difficulties.

There is a solution. The cultural mapping/intercultural exchange principles delineated throughout the text can be applied in a reverse manner. Currently employed ethnically diverse staff members can be trained and assisted to understand the mainstream U.S. cultural group orientations they encounter. English-speaking cultural formats are amenable to a cultural mapping analysis. Unfortunately, this theme is much more complex than can be accommodated within the present text, as it requires its own treatment. For the present, therefore, those professionals and providers charged with the training responsibilities for ethnically diverse personnel within their organizations might consider adapting the cultural mapping technology to develop culturally compatible educational and training formats. A working bridge to ethnically diverse aides or paraprofessionals, and other staff working in dementia-care settings, can be built. For example, the training content for these staff could be put into culture-fair contexts responsive to the diverse staff members' linguistic, interactional, and value-normative outlooks. Regrettably, the topic cannot receive the comprehensive discussion it needs within this specific narrative.

Intercultural Engagement and Dementia Research

Dementia research undertakings have not been singled out for specific mention, although Cases 5.2, 11.4, and 13.2, as well as the discussion regarding the application of cognitive assessment in Chapter 7, all have a dementia research activity origin. The discussion in the Preface indicated that many aspects of the cultural mapping formulation are likewise applicable to field and clinical research undertakings seeking to engage ethnoculturally diverse populations. There are points where research and dementia-care interests converge. Clinical trials and field studies, just like dementia-care organizations, will need to seek out, engage, and recruit ethnically diverse subjects. Both sets of efforts will need to be accompanied by culturally compatible relationship maintenance strategies. Still, there are a number of key methodological and data analysis issues that require cross-cultural attention. These include: (a) the design and subsequent application of assessment instruments to ethnically diverse populations, (b) the design and implementation of research protocols—especially those that relate to the differential diagnostic evaluation of dementing illness to different ethnocultural groups, and (c) the paradigms that are applied to the analysis of data drawn from ethnically diverse populations where cultural findings may be sometimes missed by the non-culturally attuned researcher. Admittedly, there are differences between the research and service-delivery fields centering around the manner in which the information is gathered and used.

This research agenda is therefore open for consideration; however, the issues are so extensive that they warrant their own separate treatment—a task that is not feasible within the present discussion.

Ethnopharmacology

An additional area to consider within the overall dementia-care cultural mapping/ intercultural engagement arena is the emerging findings related to *ethnopharmacology*. Some of the research undertaken has related to specific Asian subgroups (Lin et al., 1989; Lin, Poland, Smith, Strickland, & Mendoza, 1991; Lin & Shen, 1991), to African Americans (Strickland et al., 1991), and to Hispanics and American Indians/ Native Americans (R. Mendoza, Smith, Poland, Lin, & Strickland, 1991). Although the preliminary information is not directly related to dementing illness, the findings are nonetheless provocative as to the use of both psychotropic and neuroleptic medications with ethnically diverse populations with reference to both their pharmaco-dynamic and pharmacokinetic properties (Lin, Poland, & Lesser, 1986). For example, psychopharmacological researchers in the area of dementing illness in general have indicated a need for careful monitoring of the use of neuroleptics (Tune, Steele, & Cooper, 1991) and antipsychotics (Phillipson et al., 1990) with the management of behavioral symptoms among the mainstream culture group.

Given these initial findings, the cultural mapping model would indicate that dementia-care practitioners take into account what may be known about ethno-pharmacology and the ethnicity of the dementia-affected client when considering recommendations for medications. As with other themes touched on in this portion of the discussion, the topic of ethnopharmacology is much more extensive than can be delineated here beyond its identification as an important facet of cross-cultural dementia assessment and intervention.

Brief Addendum to Cultural Broker Role

Cultural brokers have been suggested as a vital adjunct to extending dementia care-services to ethnically diverse populations. The manner in which individual profession-als or providers can both identify and link to the brokers has been detailed throughout the discussion, especially in Chapter 11. The potential special role of cultural brokers in dementia care as the bilingual/bicultural member of a bicultural-pair has especially been highlighted. This role can quite possibly extend the effectiveness of the mono-cultural, English-speaking practitioner in quite helpful ways to ethnically diverse cli-ents being targeted for services. With these potentialities noted it might be important to review a number of overarching considerations regarding cultural brokers and dementia care.

First, cultural brokers are not being proposed as the panacea for extending dementia-care services to ethnoculturally diverse populations. As delineated in Chapter 10 and elsewhere, both the organization and individual practitioners have the core responsibility to move the dementia-care field ahead to become ethnoculturally relevant. Moreover, as has been previously indicated, many cultural brokers who will be encountered will have both the motivation to link their ethnic group clientele with services and the indigenous skill to move biculturally; however, they will not be dementia-care specialists. Indeed, some will be, but many will be coming from other health care and community concern areas.

Second, there are many types of cultural brokers. Some are more drawn to direct client services; others will be oriented to community organizing and advocacy. These natural career threads will need to be identified and addressed so as to effect the maximum productivity from their contributions. Professionals and providers come with many different skills, which the organization tries to match to its array of service delivery. This matching process needs to be extended to the broker recruitment and engagement effort as well.

Third, cultural brokers have a wide range of educational backgrounds. The cultural broker cadre from any single ethnically diverse group can range from an individual with little or no formal schooling to individuals with research and or medical doctorates. There are any number of degreed individuals who can also serve as *confianza-oriented* (see Chapter 11, mutualistically-oriented) resource distribution cultural brokers to their own ethnic group as well as to persons of mainstream cultural background. One should not look at cultural brokers simply as community residents. Professionals as well as indigenous peoples can fill the role.

Fourth, cultural brokers need not necessarily have been born within the ethnic group to which they broker. There is the distinct possibility that persons of Euro-Anglo ethnic heritage can become cultural brokers, apart from their participation in bicultural-pair teams. Admittedly, this is as yet a somewhat rare phenomena; however, a person originally of a Euro-Anglo English-speaking heritage can become bilingual and bicultural. There are instances of this occurring in the dementia care arena where the Euro-Anglo ethnic individual has: (a) learned the language and communicational approaches preferred by a specific ethnic group; (b) acquired a living understanding of the customs and preferred interactional styles of a specific ethnic group—that is, the individual has learned the cultural rapport and trust-building dynamics of the specific ethnic group; and (c) the person has internalized the cultural values of a specific ethnic group. The proof of the cultural synchrony of the individuals who have taken these steps is the fact that they are successfully accepted by the family members and others from the specific ethnic group to which they have chosen to relate.

It is recognized that this is a difficult idea, especially at a time when so much interaction between different ethnic groups is so politically charged. However, the central concern remains that of meeting the needs of dementia-affected elders and their caregivers who are overwhelmed by the progressive deterioration and mounting needs of the individual who has the dementing condition. Politics and conflicts aside, when considering dementia-care options, the door should not be closed to the possibility just discussed wherein persons of Euro Anglo and other mainstream backgrounds can become interethnic cultural brokers. The criteria for determining the effectiveness of this latter type of cultural broker should be the cultural competence of the individual, the acceptance of the person by the ethnically diverse family members, and role performance consistency over time.

FINAL END NOTE

Individual professionals and providers, as well as some dementia-care organizations throughout the field of dementing illness, may have a strong interest in moving ahead to offer their services across cultures. This interest should be fostered. There are approaches that can be used to develop intercultural capabilities within the dementia-care sector of services. For example, most organizations have some discretionary funds. These funds, however modest in scope, could be directed toward enhancing the organization's own internal intercultural engagement knowledge and skills. The people in the organization who are responsible for training in dementia care can rethink the use of existing teaching resources to build in a program that emphasizes cross-cultural dementia-care competencies. For instance, considerable use can be made of those individual professionals and providers at the direct-service level of the dementia-care field who have become interculturally capable. They could become part of the organization's complement of in-service training personnel.

The organizational rethinking could also come in the form of infusing cultural mapping/intercultural engagement principles into the existing practices of dementia-care agencies. Professionals and providers, as well as their parent organizations, do not need to wait for the ideas to come from the formal training programs of the different professions. The organization's directors, managers, and line staff can catch up with the changes taking place by means of redirecting their internal priorities and the available resources they command.

Agency and ethically diverse community linkages can be very quickly implemented. There is no reason why, with careful planning, the dementia-care service organization cannot begin to establish working relationships with the representatives of ethnically diverse populations and the infrastructure of indigenous agencies serving them. Also, through the use of existing information-dissemination channels, be these the Internet or formal print, audio, or visual media, dementia-care organizations can reach culturally diverse populations. The success attained can be widely disseminated through professional and provider circles.

References

Adams, J. P. (1980). Service arrangements preferred by minority elderly: A cross-cultural survey. *Journal of Gerontological Social Work, 3,* 39–56.

Adult literacy in America. (1993). Washington, DC: National Center for Education Statistics, U.S. Department of Education.

Advisory Panel on Alzheimer's Disease. (1993). *Fourth report of the Advisory Panel on Alzheimer's Disease, 1992* (NIH Publication No. 95-3520). Washington, DC: U.S. Government Printing Office.

Agar, M. (1994). The intercultural frame. *International Journal of Intercultural Relations, 18,* 221–237.

Alston, R. J., & Mngadi, S. (1992). The interaction between disability status and the African American experience: Implications for rehabilitation counseling. *Journal of Applied Rehabilitation Counseling, 23,* 12–15.

Alzheimer's: A family affair [videotape]. (1990). Washington, DC: Howard University, National Institute on Aging, and WHMM.

Alzheimer's Association. (1995). *The ten warning signs of Alzheimer's disease.* Chicago: Author.

Alzheimer's Cross Cultural Research and Development. (1992). (1) *Orientación a la enfermedad de Alzheimer* [video]; (2) *Sevicios y cuidados a largo plazo* [video]; (3) *¿Que le pasa al abuelito?* [a fotonovela]; (4) *Unodos en la lucha* [a fotonovela]. San Diego, CA: Author. [Developed for the Alzheimer's Association.]

Alzheimer's Disease and Related Disorders Association. (1994). *Multicultural outreach program manual.* Chicago: Author.

Anderson, J. (1997). *Social work with groups: A process model.* White Plains, NY: Longmans.

Anderson, N. B., & Cohen, H. J. (1989). Health status and aged minorities: Directions for clinical research. *Journal of Gerontology: Medical Sciences, 44,* M1–2.

Arrow Sciences of Mandex, Inc. (1987). *Strategies for diffusing health information to minority populations.* Springfield, VA: NTIS No. PB 85160497 HAS.

Anthony, J. C., Le Resche, L., Naiz, U., von Koroff, M. R., & Folstein, M. F. (1982). Limits of the Mini Mental State as a screening test for dementia and delirium among hospital patients. *Psychological Medicine, 12,* 397–408.

Applewhite, S. R., Wong, P., & Daly, J. M. (1991). Service approaches and issues in Hispanic agencies. *Administration and Policy in Mental Health, 19,* 27–37.

Arámbula, G. (1992). Acquired neurological disabilities in Hispanic adults. In H. Langdon & L-I. L. Cheng (Eds.), *Hispanic children and adults with communication disorders: Assessment and intervention* (pp. 373–406). Gaithersburg, MD: Aspen.

Aranda, M. P. (1987). *Siempre viva [Always with us;* videotape]. Los Angeles: CALMECAC.

Aranda, M. P. (Producer, Director). (1990). Culture-friendly services for Latino elders. *Generations, 14,* 55–57.

Aranda, M. P. & Knight, B. G. (1997). The influence of ethnicity and culture on the caregiver stress and coping process: A sociocultural review and analysis. *Gerontologist, 37,* 342–354.

Arean, P., & Gallagher-Thompson, D. (1996). Issues and recommendations for the recruitment and retention of older ethnic minority adults into clinical research. *Journal of Consulting and Clinical Psychology, 64,* 875–880.

Bahr, H. M., Chadwick, B. A., & Stauss, J. H. (1979). *American ethnicity.* Lexington, MA: D. C. Heath.

Baker, F. M. (1988). Dementing illness and black Americans. In J. Jackson (Ed.), *Black American elderly* (pp. 215–233). New York: Springer.

Banks, S. P. (1995). *Multicultural public relations: A social interpretive approach.* Thousand Oaks, CA: Sage.

Barressi, C. M., & Mennon, G. (1990). Diversity in black family caregiving. In M. S. Harper (Ed.), *Minority aging: Essential curricula content for selected health and allied professions* (pp. 297–311; DHHS Publication No. HRS PDV-904). Washington, DC: U.S. Government Printing Office.

Bates, A., & Babchuck, N. (1961). The primary group: A reappraisal. *Sociological Quarterly, 11,* 181–191.

Bedolla, M. A. (1995). Principles of medical ethics and their application to Mexican-American elderly patients. *Clinics in Geriatric Medicine, 11,* 131–137.

Berghe, P. V. D. (1972). *Intergroup relations: Sociological perspectives.* New York: Basic Books.

Berlin, E., & Fowkes, W. (1983). A teaching framework for cross-cultural health care: Application in family practice. *Western Journal of Medicine, 139,* 934–938.

Betancourt, H., & Regeser López, S. (1993). The study of culture, ethnicity, and race in American psychology. *American Psychologist, 48,* 629–637.

Biegel, D. E., Shore, B. K., & Gordon, E. (1982). *Building support networks for the elderly: Theory and applications.* Beverly Hills, CA: Sage.

Bird, H. R., Canino, G., & Shrout, P. E. (1987). Use of the Mini-Mental State Examination in a probability sample of a Hispanic population. *Journal of Nervous and Mental Disease, 175,* 731–737.

Birkel, R. C., & Reppucci, N. D. (1983). Social networks, information-seeking, and utilization of services. *American Journal of Community Psychology, 11,* 185–205.

Bochner, S. (Ed.). (1982). *Cultures in contact.* New York: Pergamon Press.

Borrini, B., Dall'Ora, P., Della Sala, S., Marinelli, L., & Spinnler, H. (1989). Autobiographical memory: Sensitivity to age and education of a standardized enquiry. *Psychological Medicine, 19,* 215–224.

Boston, P. (1992). Understanding cultural differences through family assessment. *Journal of Cancer Education, 7*(3), 261–266.

Braun, K. L., Takamura, J. C., Forman, S., Sasaki, P. A., & Meininger, L. (1995). Developing and testing outreach materials on Alzheimer's disease for Asian and Pacific Islander Americans. *The Gerontologist, 35,* 125–126.

Brislin, R. (1993). *Understanding culture's influence on behavior.* Orlando, FL: Harcourt Brace Jovanovich.

Brislin, R. W., & Yoshida, T. (1994). *Improving intercultural interactions: Modules for cross-cultural training programs.* Thousand Oaks, CA: Sage.

Brownlee, A. T. (1978). *Community, culture, and care: A cross-cultural guide for health workers.* St. Louis, MO: C. V. Mosby.

Buchanan, A. & Brock, D. W. (1986). Deciding for others. *The Milbank Quarterly, 64* (Suppl. 2), 17–94.

Burns, B. (1992). Hispanic caregiver project uses cognitive therapy techniques. *Aging, 363/364,* 38–39.

Burton, L., Kasper, J., Shore, A., Cagney, C., LaVeist, T., Cubbin, C., & German, P. (1995). The structure of informal care: Are there differences by race? *The Gerontologist, 6,* 744–752.

Butcher, J. N. (1982). Cross-cultural research methods in clinical psychology. In P. C. Kendall & J. N. Butcher (Eds.), *Handbook of research methods in clinical psychology* (pp. 272–308). New York: Wiley.

Cancelmo, J. A, Millan, F., & Vazquez, C. I. (1990). Culture and symptomatology: The role of personal meaning in diagnosis and treatment: A case study. *American Journal of Psychoanalysis, 50,* 137–149.

Canino, I. A., Rubio-Stipic, M., Canino, G., & Escobar, J. I. (1992). Functional somatic symptoms: A cross-ethnic comparison. *American Journal of Orthopsychiatry, 62,* 605–612.

Chee, P., & Kane, R. (1983). Cultural factors affecting nursing home care for minorities: A study of Black American and Japanese American groups. *Journal of the American Geriatrics Society, 31,* 109–112.

Cheng, L-I. L. (1987). *Assessing Asian language performance: Guidelines for evaluating limited English language students.* Rockville, MD: Aspen.

Christensen, H., & Jorm, A. F. (1992). Effect of premorbid intelligence on the Mini-Mental State and the IQCODE. *International Journal of Geriatric Psychiatry, 7,* 159–160.

Christman, N. J. (1977). The health seeking process: An approach to the natural history of illness. *Culture, Medicine, and Psychiatry, 1,* 351–377.

Chu, I. (1991). Family care of the elderly with dementia in Hong Kong. *International Social Work, 34,* 365–372.

Clark, M., & Anderson, B. G. (1967). *Culture and aging.* Springfield, IL: Charles C Thomas.

Cooley, C. (1909). *Social organization.* New York: Scribner.

Cooley, R. C., Ostendorf, D., & Bickerto, D. (1976). Outreach services for elderly Native Americans. *Social Work, 21,* 151–153.

Cowgill, D. O. (1986). *Aging around the world.* Belmont, CA: Wadsworth.

Cox, C. (1993). Service needs and interests: A comparison of African American and white caregivers seeking Alzheimer assistance. *American Journal of Alzheimer's Care and Related Disorders Research, 8,* 33–40.

Cox, C., & Monk, A. (1990). Minority caregivers of dementia victims: A comparison of black and Hispanic families. *Journal of Applied Gerontology, 29,* 340–354.

Cox, C., & Monk, A. (1993). Hispanic culture and family care of Alzheimer's patients. *Health and Social Work, 18,* 92–99.

Cross, A. (1996). Working with American Indian elders in the city: Reflections of an American Indian social worker. In G. Yeo & D. Gallagher-Thompson (Eds.), *Ethnicity and the dementias* (pp. 183–185). Washington, DC: Taylor and Francis.

Cuellar, I., Arnold, B., & Maldonado, R. (1995). Acculuration rating scale for Mexican Americans–II: A revision of the original ARSMA Scale. *Hispanic Journal of Behavioral Sciences, 17,* 275–304.

Cuellar, I., Harris, L. C., & Jasso, R. (1980). An acculturation scale for Mexican American normal and clinical populations. *Hispanic Journal of Behavioral Sciences, 2,* 199–207.

Culture and caregiving. (1992). *Aging, 363/364,* 29–31.

Cunningham, C. V. (1991–1992). Reaching minority communities: Factors impacting on success. *Journal of Gerontological Social Work, 17–18,* 125–135.

Cushner, K., & Brislin, R. W. (1996). *Intercultural interactions: A practical guide* (2nd ed.). Thousand Oaks, CA: Sage.

Day, J. C. (1995). *Population projections of the United States by age, sex, race, and Hispanic origin, 1995–2050* (U.S. Bureau of the Census Current Population Report No. P25-1130). Washington, DC: U.S. Government Printing Office.

Draguns, J. G. (1996). Humanly universal and culturally distinctive: Charting the course of cultural counseling. In P. B. Pedersen, J. G. Draguns, W. L. Lonner, & J. E. Trimble (Eds.), *Counseling cross cultures* (pp. 1–20). Thousand Oaks, CA: Sage Publications.

DuBrin, A. J. (1974). *Fundamentals of organizational behavior.* New York: Pergamon Press, Inc.

Dungee-Anderson, D., & Beckett, J. O. (1992). Alzheimer's disease in African American and white families: A clinical analysis. *Smith College Studies in Social Work, 62,* 155–168.

Ekman, S. L., Wahlin, T. B., Norberg, A., & Winblad, B. (1993). Relationship between bilingual demented immigrants and bilingual/monolingual caregivers. *International Journal of Aging and Human Development, 37*(1), 37–57.

Elliot, K. S., Di Minno, M., Lam, D., & Mei Tu, A. (1996). Working with Chinese families in the context of dementia. In G. Yeo & D. Gallagher-Thompson (Eds.), *Ethnicity and the dementias* (pp. 189–108). Washington, DC: Taylor and Francis.

Eribes, R. A., & Bradley-Rawls, M. (1978). The underutilization of nursing home facilities by Mexican-American elderly in the Southwest. *The Gerontologist, 18,* 363–371.

Escobar, J. I., Burnam, A., Karno, M., Forsythe, A., Lansverk, J., & Golding, J. M. (1986). Use of the Mini-Mental State Examination (MMSE) in a community population of mixed ethnicity. *Journal of Nervous and Mental Disease, 174,* 607–614.

Evans, D. A. (1992). Alzheimer's disease: Where will we find the etiologic clues? Challenges and opportunities in cross-cultural studies. *Ethnicity and Disease, 2,* 321–375.

Farley, J. E. (1995). *Majority–minority relations.* Englewood Cliffs, NJ: Prentice Hall.

Farris, E. (1932). The primary group. *American Journal of Sociology, 1,* 41–55.

Fegurgur, M. K. (1995). *A comparative study of Anglo, Hispanic, and Chamorro caregivers of dementia-affected elders.* Unpublished master's thesis, San Diego State University.

Fellin, P. (1995). *The community and the social worker* (2nd ed.). Itasca, IL: F. E. Peacock.

Festinger, L. (1962). *A theory of cognitive dissonance.* Stanford, CA: Stanford University Press.

Fine, M. G. (1995). *Building successful multicultural organizations.* Westport, CT: Quorum Books.

Flan, E. (1991). The Appalachian voice. In *The annual editions series* (pp. 130–137). Guilford, CT: Dushkin.

Folstein, M. F., Folstein, S. A., & McHough, P. R. (1975). Mini Mental State: A practical method for grading the cognitive state of patients for the clinician. *Journal of Psychiatric Research, 12,* 189–198.

Fredman, L., Daly, M. P., & Lazur, A. M. (1995). Burden among white and black caregivers to elderly adults. *Journal of Gerontology: Social Sciences, 50B,* S110–S118.

Gaines, A. D. (1988–1989). Alzheimer's disease in the context of black (Southern) culture. *Health Matrix, 6,* 33–38.

Gallagher-Thompson, D., Arguello, D., Johnson, C., Moorehead, R. S., & Polich, T. M. (1992). *Cmo controlar la frustracin: Una clase para el cuidadante* [Controlling your frustration: A clause for caregivers]. Palo Alto, CA: Department of Veterans Affairs Medical Center.

Gallagher-Thompson, D., Moorehead, R. S., Plich, T. M., Arguello, D., Johnson, C., Rodriguez, V., & Meyer, M. (1994). A comparison of outreach strategies for Hispanic caregivers of Alzheimer's victims. *Clinical Gerontologist, 15,* 57–63.

Gallagher-Thompson, D., Talamantes, M., Ramirez, R., & Valverde, R. (1996). Service delivery issues and recommendations for working with the Mexican American family. In G. Yeo & D. Gallagher-Thompson (Eds.), *Ethnicity and the dementias* (pp. 137–152). Washington, DC: Taylor and Francis.

Gelfand, D. E., & Fandetti, D. V. (1980). Suburban and urban white ethnics: Attitudes towards care of the aged. *The Gerontologist, 20,* 588–594.

Gentile, M. C. (Ed.). (1994). *Differences that work: Organizational excellence through diversity.* Boston: Harvard Business School.

Germaine, C. B. (1991). *Human behavior and the social environment: An ecological view.* New York: Columbia University Press.

Gerontological Society of America. (1991). *Minority elders: Longevity, economics, and health..* Washington, DC: Author.

Gibson, R. C. (1989). Minority aging research: Opportunity and challenge. *Journal of Gerontology: Social Sciences, 44,* S2–S3.

Gonzalez, E., Gitlin, L., & Lyons, K. J. (1995). Review of the literature on African American caregivers of individuals with dementia. *Journal of Cultural Diversity, 2,* 40–48.

Goodman, C. (1989). *Reaching out to a multicultural community: Challenges for adult day care centers.* Sacramento, CA: California Department of Aging, Alzheimer's/Mental Health Branch.

Grabowski, J-A., & Franz, T. T. (1992–1993). Latinos and Anglos: Cultural experiences of grief intensity. *OMEGA, 24,* 273–285.

Graham, J. L. (1993). The Japanese negotiation style: Characteristics of a distinct approach. *Negotiation Journal, 9,* 123–140.

Gratton, B., & Wilson, V. (1988). Family support systems and minority elderly: A cautionary analysis. *Journal of Gerontological Social Work, 13,* 81–93.

Green, V. (1987). Underlying issues of diversity in the study of aging blacks. In H. Strange & M. Teitelbaum (Eds.), *Aging and cultural diversity: New directions and annotated bibliography* (pp. 101–130). Westport, CT: Bergin & Garvey.

Green, V. L., & Monohan, D. J. (1984). Comparative utilization of community based long term care services by Hispanic and Anglo elderly in a case management system. *Journal of Gerontology, 39,* 730–735.

Greer, C. (1974). *Divided society: The ethnic experience in America.* New York: Basic Books.

Grosjean, F. (1982). *Life with two languages.* Cambridge, MA: Harvard University Press.

Gudykunst, W. B. (1994). *Bridging differences: Effective intergroup communications* (2nd ed.). Newbury Park, CA: Sage.

Haddock, R. L., & Santos, J. V. (1992). Are the endemic motor neuron diseases of Guam really disappearing? *Southeast Journal of Tropical Medicine and Public Health, 28,* 278–281.

Haley, W., West, W., Wadley, V., White, F., Barret, J., Ford, G., Harrell, L., & Roth, D. (1995). Psychological, social and health impact of caregiving: A comparison of black and white dementia caregivers and non-caregivers. *Psychology and Aging, 10,* 540–552.

Ham, M. (1987). How to assess the needs of minorities. *Provider, 6,* 45, 51.

Hamayan, E.V., & Damico, J. S (1991). *Limiting bias in the assessment of bilingual students.* Austin, TX: Pro-Ed.

Hanna, W. J., & Rogovsky, E. (1992). On the situation of African-American women with physical disabilities. *Journal of Applied Rehabilitation Counseling, 23,* 39–45.

Hardcastle, D. A., Wencour, S., & Powers, P. R. (1997). *Community practice: Theories and skills for social workers.* New York: Oxford University Press.

Harper, K. V., & Lanz, J. (1996). *Cross-cultural practice: Social work with diverse populations.* Chicago: Lyceum Books.

Harris, P. R., & Moran, R. T. (1987). *Managing cultural differences: High performance strategies for today's global manager.* Houston, TX: Gulf.

Havenaar, J. M. (1990). Psychotherapy: Healing by culture. *Psychotherapy and Psychosomatics, 53,* 8–18.

Heisel, M., & Larson, G. (1984). Literacy and the social milieu: Behavior and the black elderly. *Adult Education Quarterly, 34,* 63–70.

Helms, J. E. (1992). Why is there no study of cultural equivalence in standardized cognitive ability testing? *American Psychologist, XX,* 1083–1099.

Henderson, J. N. (1987). Caregiving in culturally diverse populations. *Seminars in Speech and Language, 15,* 216–225.

Henderson, J. N. (1990a). Alzheimer's disease in a cultural context. In J. Sokolovsky (Ed.), *The cultural context of aging: Worldwide perspectives* (pp. 315–330). Westport, CT: Bergin & Garvey.

Henderson, J. N. (1990b). Anthropology, health and aging. In R. L. Rubenstein (Ed.), *Anthropology and aging: Comprehensive reviews* (pp. 39–68). Boston: Kluwer Academic.

Henderson, J. N. (1992). The power of support: Alzheimer's disease support groups for minority families. *Aging, 263/264,* 24–28.

Henderson, J. N. (1996). Cultural dynamics in a Cuban and Puerto Rican population in the United States. In G. Yeo & D. Gallagher-Thompson (Eds.), *Ethnicity and dementia* (pp. 153–166). Washington, DC: Taylor and Francis.

Henderson, J. N., & Gutierrez-Mayka, M. (1992). Ethnocultural themes in caregiving to Alzheimer's disease patients in Hispanic families. *Clinical Gerontologist, 11,* 59–74.

Henderson, J. N., Gutierrez-Mayka, M., Garcia, J., & Boyd, S. (1993). A model for Alzheimer's disease support group development in African-American and Hispanic populations. *The Gerontologist, 33,* 409–414.

Hendrie, H. C., Hall, K. S., Pillay, N., Rodgers, D., Prince, C., Norton, J., Brittain, H., Nath, A., Blue, A., Kaufert, J., Shelton, P., Postl, B., & Osuntokun, B. (1993). Alzheimer's disease is rare among the Cree. *International Geriatrics, 5,* 5–13.

Hendrie, H. C., Osuntokun, B. O., Hall, K. S., Ogunniyi, A. O., Hui, S. L., Unverzagt, F. W., Gureje, O., Rodenberg, C. A., Baiyewu, O., Musick, B. S., Adeyinka, A., Farlow, M. R., Oluwole, S. O., Class, C. A., Komolafe, O., Brashear, A., & Burdine, V. (1995). Prevalence of Alzheimer's disease and dementia in two communities: Nigerian Africans, and African Americans. *American Journal of Psychiatry, 152,* 1485–1492.

Hennessy, C. H., & John, J. R. (1995). Interpretation of burden among Pueblo Indian caregivers. *Journal of Aging Studies, 9,* 215–229.

Hepworth, D. H., & Larsen, J. A. (1993). *Direct social work practice: Theory and skills* (4th ed.). Pacific Grove, CA: Brooks/Cole.

Herskovits, M. J. (1973). *Cultural relativism: Perspectives on cultural pluralism.* New York: Vintage Books.

Heyman, A., Fillenbaum, G., Prosnitz, B., Raiford, K., Burchett, B., & Clark, C. (1991). Estimated prevalence of dementia among elderly black and white community residents. *Archives of Neurology, 48,* 594–598.

Hill, L. R., Klauber, M. R., Salmon, D. P., Yu, E. S. U., Liu, W. T., Zhang, M., & Katzman, R. (1993). Functional status, education, and diagnosis of dementia in the Shanghai survey. *Neurology, 43,* 138–145.

Himes, C. L., Hogan, D. P., & Eggebeen, D. J. (1996). Living arrangements of minority elders. *Journal of Gerontology: Social Sciences, 51B,* S42–S48.

Hines, P. M., Garcia-Preto, N., McGoldrick, M., Almeida, R., & Weltman, S. (1992). Intergenerational relationships across cultures. *Journal of Contemporary Human Services, 73,* 323–338.

Hinkle, L. E., & Wolff, H. G. (1957). The nature of man's adaptation to his total environment and the relation of this to illness. *Archives of Internal Medicine, 99,* 442–461.

Hinrichen, G. A., & Ramirez, M. (1992). Black and white dementia caregivers: A comparison of their adaptation, adjustment, and service utilization. *The Gerontologist, 32,* 375–381.

Holmes, D., Holmes, M., Steinback, L., Hausner, T., & Rocheleau, B. (1979). The use of community-based services in long-term care by older minority persons. *The Gerontologist, 19,* 379–397.

Holmes, D., Teresi, J., & Holmes, M. (1981). Differences among blacks and whites in knowledge about and attitudes towards long-term care services. *Quarterly Contact, 4,* 1, 5.

Holzer, III, C. E., Shea, B. M., Swanson, J. W., Leaf, P. J., Myers, J. K., George, L., Weissman, M. M., & Bedmarski, P. (1986). The increased risk for specific psychiatric disorders among persons of low socioeconomic status. *American Journal of Social Psychiatry, 6,* 260–270.

Holzer, III, C. E., Tischer, G. L., Leaf, P. J., & Myers, J. K. (1984). An epidemiologic assessment of cognitive impairment in a community population. *Research Communication in Mental Health, 4,* 3–32.

Homma, A., Ishii, T., & Niina, R. (1994). Relationship of behavioral complications and severity of dementia in Japanese elderly persons with dementia. *Alzheimer Disease and Associated Disorders, 8*(Suppl. 3), 46–53.

Hovaguimian, T., Henderson, S., Katchaturian, Z., & Orley, J. (Eds.). (1989). *The classification and diagnosis of Alzheimer's disease: An international perspective.* Toronto: Hogrefe & Huber.

Hraba, J. (1994). *American ethnicity.* Itaska, IL: F. E. Peacock.

Hyltenstam, K., & Obler, L. K. (1989). *Bilingualism across the lifespan: Aspects of acquisition, maturity, and loss.* New York: Cambridge University Press.

Institute for Community Research. (1992). *Educational materials and innovative dissemination strategies: Alzheimer's disease among Puerto Rican elderly.* Hartfort, CA: Author.

Ivey, A. E. (1994). *Intentional counseling: Facilitating client development in a multicultural society* (3rd ed.). Pacific Grove, CA: Brooks/Cole.

Jackson, H. (1983). Geriatric patients of minority groups. *Psychiatric Opinion, 11,* 14–19.

Jackson, J. S., Burns, C., & Gibson, R. (1992). An overview of geriatric care in ethnic and racial minority groups. In E. Calkins, P. J. Davis, A. B. Ford, & P. J. Katz (Eds.), *Practice of geriatrics* (2nd ed., pp. 57–64). Philadelphia: W. B. Saunders.

Jecker, N. S., Carrese, J. A., & Pearlman, R. A. (1995). Caring for patients in cross-cultural settings. *Hastings Center Report, 25,* 6–14.

Jenkins, J. H., & Karno, M. (1992). The meaning of expressed emotion: Theoretical issues raised by cross-cultural research. *American Journal of Psychiatry, 149,* 9–21.

Kapp, M. B. (1994). Proxy decision making in Alzheimer disease research: Durable powers of attorney, guardianship, and other alternatives. *Alzheimer Disease and Associated Disorders, 8* (Suppl. 4), 28–37.

Katzman, R., Zhang, M., Ouang, Y-Q., Wang, Z., Liu, W., Yu, E., Wong, S-C., Salmon, D. P., & Grant, I. A. (1988). A Chinese version of the Mini-Mental State Examination: Impact of illiteracy in a Shanghai dementia survey. *Journal of Clinical Epidemiology, 41,* 971–978.

Kawaga-Singer, M. (1994). Diverse cultural beliefs and practices about death and dying in the elderly. *Gerontology and Geriatrics Education, 15*(1), 101–116.

Keith, J., Fry, C. L., Glascock, A. P., Ikels, C., Dickerson-Putman, J., Harpending, H. C., & Draper, P. (1994). *The aging experience: Diversity and commonality across cultures.* Thousand Oaks, CA: Sage.

Kessler, R. C., & Neighbors, H. W. (1986). A new perspective on the relationships among race, social class, and psychological distress. *Journal of Health and Social Behavior, 27,* 107–115.

Kim, K. C., Kim, S., & Hurh, W. M. (1991). Filial piety and intergenerational relationships in Korean immigrant families. *International Journal of Aging and Human Development, 33,* 233–245.

Kinneman, J. A. (1947). *The community in American society.* New York: Appleton–Century–Crofts.

Kleinman, A. M. (1977). Depression, somatization, and the new cross-cultural psychiatry. *Social Science and Medicine, 11,* 3–10.

Kleinman, A. (1980). *Patient and healers in the context of culture: An exploration of the borderland between anthropology, medicine, and psychiatry.* Berkeley: University of California Press.

Kleinman, A. M. (1986a). Concepts and a model for the comparison of medical systems as cultural systems. In C. Currer & M. Stacey (Eds.), *Concepts of health and illness and disease* (pp. 27–50). New York: Guilford Press.

Kleinman, A. M. (1986b). *Social origins of distress and disease: Depression, neurasthenia, and pain in modern China.* New Haven, CT: Yale University Press.

Kluckhohn, C. (1965). *Mirror for man: A survey of human behavior and social attitudes.* Greenwich, CT: Fawcett.

Kobayashi, S., Masaki, H., & Noguchi, M. (1993). Developmental processes: Family caregivers of demented Japanese. *Journal of Gerontological Nursing, 19,* 7–12.

Kramer, J. B. (1991). Urban American Indian aging. *Journal of Cross-Cultural Gerontology, 6,* 205–217.

Kramer, J. B. (1992a). Health and aging of urban American Indians. *Western Journal of Medicine, 157,* 281–285.

Kramer, J. B. (1992b). Serving American elderly in cities: An invisible minority. *Aging, 363/364,* 48–51.

Kramer, J. B. (1996). Dementia and American Indian populations. In G.Yeo & D. Gallagher-Thompson (Eds.), *Ethnicity and the dementias* (pp. 175–181). Washington, DC: Taylor and Francis.

Krause, N., & Wray, L. A. (1991). Psychological correlates of health and illness among minority elders. *Generations, 15,* 25–30.

Kromkowski, J. A. (Ed.). (1993–1994). *Race and ethnic relations, 93–94.* Guilford, CT: Dushkin.

Kwanzaa Information Center. (1997). http://www.melanet.com/kwanzaa/#background.

Larson, E. B., & Imai, Y. (1996). An overview of dementia and ethnicity with special emphasis on the epidemiology of dementia. In G. Yeo & D. Gallagher-Thompson (Eds.), *Ethnicity and the dementias* (pp. 9–20). Washington, DC: Taylor & Francis.

Lavine, L., Steele, J., Wolfe, N., Calne, D. B., O'Brien, P., Williams, D. B., Kurland, L. T., & Shoenberg, B. (1991). Amyotrophic lateral sclerosis/Parkinsonism–dementia complex in Southern Guam: Is it disappearing? *Advances in Neurology, 56,* 271–285.

Lawton, M. P. (1994). Quality of life in Alzheimer's disease. *Alzheimer Disease and Associated Disorders, 8*(Suppl. 3), 138–150.

Lawton, M. P., Rajagopal, D., Brody, E., & Kleban, M. H. (1992). The dynamics of caregiving for a demented elder among black and white families. *Journal of Gerontology: Social Sciences, 47*(4), S156–S164.

LeCours, A. R., Mehler, J., Parente, M. A., Calderia, A., Cary, L., Castro, M. J., Dehaut, F., Delgado, R., Gurd, J., de Fraga, K., Jakubovitz, R., Osorio, S., Scliar Cabral, L., & Sares Junqueria, M. (1987). Illiteracy and brain damage–I: Aphasia testing of culturally contrasted populations (control subjects). *Neuropsicologia, 25,* 231–245.

Lewin, K. (1936). *Principles of topological psychology.* New York: McGraw-Hill.

Lewis, I. D., & Chavis Ausbery, M. S. (1996). African American families: Management of demented elders. In G. Yeo & D. Gallagher-Thompson (Eds.), *Ethnicity and the dementias* (pp. 225–233). Washington, DC: Taylor and Francis.

Li, G., Shen, Y. C., Chen, C. H., Zhao, Y. W., Li, S. R., & Lu, M. (1989). An epidemiological survey of age-related dementia in an urban area of Bejing. *Acta Psychiatrica Scandinavia, 79,* 557–563.

Lilienfeld, D. E., & Perl, D. P. (1994). Projected neurodegenerative disease mortality among minorities in the United States, 1990–2040. *Neuroepidemiology, 13,* 179–186.

Lin, K-M., Innui, T. S., Kleirman, A., & Womak, W. (1982). Socio-cultural determinants of the help-seeking behavior of patients with mental illness. *Journal of Nervous and Mental Disease, 170,* 78–85.

Lin, K-M., Poland, R. E., & Lesser, I. M. (1986). Ethnicity and psychopharmacology. *Culture, Medicine, and Psychiatry, 10,* 151–165.

Lin, K-M., Poland, R. E., Nuccio, I., Matsuda, K., Hathuc, N., Su, T-P., & Fu, P. (1989). Longitudinal assessment of Haloperidol doses and serum concentrations in Asian and Caucasian schizophrenic patients. *American Journal of Psychiatry, 146,* 1307–1311.

Lin, K-M., Poland, R. E., Smith, M. W., Strickland, T. L., & Mendoza, R. (1991). Pharmacokinetic and other related factors affecting psychotropic responses in Asians. *Psychopharmacology Bulletin, 27,* 427–439.

Lin, K-M., & Shen, W. W. (1991). Psychopharmacology for Southeast Asian psychiatric patients. *Journal of Nervous and Mental Disease, 179,* 346–350.

Litwak, E., & Szelenyi, R. (1969). Primary group structures and their function, kin, neighbors, and friends. *American Sociological Review, 4,* 465–481.

Liu, H. C., Lin, K. N., Tsou, H. K, Lee, K. M., Yan, S. H., Wang, S. J., & Chiang, B. N. (1991). Impact of demented patients on their family members and care-givers in Taiwan. *Neuroepidemiology, 10*(3), 143–149.

Liu, H. C., Tsou, H. K., Lin, K. N., Guo, N. W., Wang, C. L., & Chiang, B. N. (1991). Evaluation of 110 consecutive patients with dementia: A prospective study. *Acta Neurologica Scandanavia, 84,* 421–425.

Lockery, S. A. (1987). Impact of dementia within minority groups. Contractor Documents, Part 2: Economics, social science, and health services research. Conducted for: U.S. Congress, Office of Technology Assessment: Losing a Million Minds: Confronting the tragedy of Alzheimer's disease and other dementias. Springfield, VA: National Technical Information Service, U.S. Department of Commerce.

Lockery, S. A. (1991). Family and social supports: Caregiving among racial and ethnic minority elders. *Generations, 15,* 58–62.

Loftland, J., & Loftland, L. H. (1995). *Analyzing social settings: A guide to qualitative observation and analysis* (2nd ed.). Belmont, CA: Wadsworth.

Lonner, W. J. (1981). Psychological tests and intercultural counseling. In P. B. Pedersen, J. G. Draguns, W. J. Lonner, & J. E. Trimble (Eds.), *Counseling across cultures,* (pp. 275–303). Honolulu: East West Center and University of Hawaii.

Lonner, W. J., & Ibrahim, F. A. (1996). Appraisal and assessment in cross-cultural counseling. In P. B. Pedersen, J. G. Draguns, W. L. Lonner, and J. E. Trimble (Eds.), *Counseling across cultures* (pp. 293–322). Thousand Oaks, CA: Sage Publications.

Lopez, S., & Taussig, I. M. (1991). Cognitive–intellectual functioning of Spanish-speaking impaired and non-impaired elderly: Implications for culturally sensitive assessments. *Psychological Assessment, 3,* 448–454.

Lubben, J. E. (1988). Assessing social networks among elderly populations. *Family and Community Health, 11,* 42–52.

Lubben, J. E., & Becerra, R. M. (1987). Social support among black, Mexican, and Chinese elderly. In

D. E. Gelfand & C. M. Barresi (Eds.), *Ethnic dimensions of aging* (pp. 130–144). New York: Springer.

Mace, N., & Rabins, P. (1990). *Cuando el da tiene 36 horas* [The 36 hour day]. México, D.F.: Editorial Pax México.

Manson, S. M. (1989). Provider assumptions about long term-care in American Indian communities. *The Gerontologist, 29,* 355–358.

Manson, S. (1993). Long-term care of older American Indians: Challenges in the development of institutional services. In C. M. Barresi & D. E. Stull (Eds.), *Ethnic elders and long-term care* (pp. 130–143). New York: Springer.

Manubens, J. M., Martinez-Lage, J. M., Lacruz, F., Murunzabal, J., Larumbe, R., Guarch, C., Urrutia, T., Sarrasqueta, P., Martinez-Lage, P., & Rocca, W. A. (1995). Prevalence of Alzheimer's disease and other dementing disorders in Pamelova, Spain. *Neuroepidemiology, 14,* 155–164.

Manuel, R. C. (Ed.). (1982). *Minority aging: Social and social psychological issues.* Westport, CT: Greenwood Press.

Mattes, L. J., & Omark, D. R. (1984). *Speech and language assessment for the bilingual handicapped.* San Diego, CA: College Hill Press, Inc.

Mauro, R., Sato, K., & Tucker, J. (1992). The role of appraisal in human emotions: A cross-cultural study. *Journal of Personality and Social Psychology, 62,* 301–307.

Mayers, M. K. (1980). *A look at Filipino lifestyles.* Dallas, TX: Sil Museum of Anthropology.

McBride, M. R., & Parreno, H. (1996). Filipino American families and caregiving. In G. Yeo & D. Gallagher-Thompson (Eds.), *Ethnicity and the dementias* (pp. 123–135). Washington, DC: Taylor and Francis.

McDaniel, T. (1996). *Community analysis working paper.* Unpublished manuscript.

McDonald-Shoemaker, D. (1981). Navajo nursing homes: Conflict of philosophies. *Journal of Gerontological Nursing, 7,* 531–536.

McLemore, D. S. (1994). *Racial and ethnic relations in America.* Boston: Allyn & Bacon.

Mendoza, L. (1980). Hispanic helping networks: Techniques of cultural support. In R. Valle & W. Vega (Eds.), *Hispanic natural support systems: Mental health promotion perspectives* (pp. 55–63). Sacramento: State of California Department of Mental Health.

Mendoza, L. (1981a). Los servidores: Caretakers among the Hispanic elderly. *Generations, 5,* 25–26.

Mendoza, L. (1981b). *The servidor system: Policy implications for the elder Latino.* San Diego, CA: San Diego State University Center on Aging.

Mendoza, R., Smith, M.W., Poland, R. E., Lin, K-M., & Strickland, T. L. (1991). Ethnic psychopharmacology: The Hispanic and Native American perspective. *Psychopharmacology Bulletin, 27,* 449–461.

Mesquita, B., & Frijda, N. H. (1992). Cultural variations in emotions: A review. *Psychological Bulletin, 112,* 179–204.

Meyerson, M. D. (1994). Many cultures/more compassion. *Journal of Clinical Pharmacy and Therapeutics, 19,* 215–218.

Miner, S. (1995). Racial differences in family support and formal service utilization among older persons: A nonrecursive model. *Journal of Gerontology: Social Sciences, 50B,* S143–S153.

Minority elders: Longevity, economics, and health. (1991). Washington, DC: Gerontological Society of America.

Mintzer, J., Loewenstein, D., Millor, A., Flores, L., & Rainerman, A. (1992). Daughters caregiving for Hispanic and non-Hispanic Alzheimer's patients: Does ethnicity make a difference? *Community Mental Health Journal, 28,* 293–303.

Mintzer, J., & Macera, C. (1992). Prevalence of depressive symptoms among white and African American caregivers of demented patients. *American Journal of Psychiatry, 149,* 575–576.

Mintzer, J. E. (1994). Ethnicity, culture, and mental health: The long term care of ethnicity. *The American Journal of Geriatric Psychiatry, 14,* 10–12.

Mintzer, J. E., Knapp, R., Herman, K. C., Johnson, K. W., Mietert, P., & Walters, T. H. (in press). Differences in the caregiving experiences between African American and White caregivers of demented elderly patients. *Journal of Clinical Psychiatry.*

Mintzer, J. E., Macera, C., Herman, K. C., Jannarone, R. J., & Davis, D. R. (in press). Depressive symptoms in white and African-American caregivers. *Journal of Minority Aging.*

Mintzer, J. E., Nietart, P., Costa, K.,& Waid, L. R. (in press). Cross-cultural perpectives: Agitation in demented patients in the U.S. *International Psychogeriatrics.*

Mintzer, J. E., Rupert, M. P., & Herman, K. C. (in press). Caregiving for Hispanic Alzheimer patients. *American Journal of Geriatric Psychiatry.*

Mintzer, J. E., Rupert, M. P., Loewenstein, D. A., Gamez, E., Millor, A., Quinteros, R., Flores, L., Miller, M., Rainerman, A., & Eisdorfer, C. (1992). Daughters caregiving for Hispanic and non-Hispanic Alzheimer's patients: Does ethnicity make a difference? *Community Mental Health Journal, 28,* 293–303.

Montalvo, B., & Gutierrez, M. (1989). Nine assumptions for work with ethnic minority families. *Journal of Psychotherapy and the Family, 6,* 35–52.

Moore Hines, P., Garcia-Preto, N., McGoldrick, M., Almeida, R., & Wetman, S. (1992). Intergenerational relationships across cultures. *Families in Society: The Journal of Contemporary Human Services,* 323–338.

Morganthau, T. (1997, January 27). The face of the future. *Newsweek, 129*(4), 58–60.

Morrison, B. J. (1982). Sociocultural dimensions: Nursing homes and the minority aged. *Journal of Gerontological Social Work, 5,* 127–145.

Morycz, R. K., Malloy, J., Bozich, M., & Martz, P. (1987). Racial differences in family burden: Clinical implications for social work. *Journal of Gerontological Social Work, 10,* 133–154.

Mui, A. (1992). Caregiver strain among black and white daughter caregivers: A role theory perspective. *The Gerontologist, 32,* 203–212.

Mui, A. C., & Burnette, D. (1994). Longer term care use by frail elders: Is ethnicity a factor? *The Gerontologist, 34,* 190–198.

Mungas, D. (1996). The process of development of valid and reliable neuropsychological assessment measures for English- and Spanish-speaking elderly persons. In G. Yeo & D. Gallagher-Thompson (Eds.), *Ethnicity and the dementias* (pp. 33–46). Washington, DC: Taylor & Francis.

Mungas, D., Marshall, S. C., Weldon, M., Haan, M., & Reed, B. R. (1996). Age and education correction of the Mini-Mental State Examination for English- and Spanish-speaking elderly. *Neurology, 46,* 700–706.

Murden, R. A., McRae, T. D., Kaner, S., & Buckman, M. E. (1991). Mini-Mental State Exam scores vary with education in blacks and whites. *American Geriatrics Society, 39,* 149–155.

Murdock, S. H., Schwartz, D. F., & Hwang, S. (1980). The effects of socioeconomic characteristics and off-reservation contacts on the service awareness and usage patterns of elderly Native Americans. *Long Term Care and Health Services Administration Quarterly, 4,* 64–76.

Mutran, E. (1985). Intergenerational family support among blacks and whites: Response to culture or to socioeconomic differences? *Journal of Gerontology, 40,* 382–389.

Nakano, K. (1991). Coping strategies and psychological symptoms in a Japanese sample. *Journal of Clinical Psychology, 47,* 346–350.

Naparastek, A. J., Beigel, D. E., & Spiro, H. R. (1982). *Neighborhood networks for humane mental health care.* New York: Plenum.

Netting, F. E., Kettner, P. M., & McMurtry, S. L. (1993). *Social work macropractice.* White Plains, NY: Longman.

Ng, L. L. (1994). Psychiatry in dementia. *Singapore Medical Journal, 35*(1), 96–99.

Novak, F. (1974). Home nursing care program on an Indian reservation. *Public Health Reports, 89,* 545–550.

Novak, M. (1972). *The rise of the unmeltable ethnics.* New York: Macmillan.

Nunes, T. (1995). Cultural practices and the conception of individual differences: Theoretical and empirical considerations. *New Directions for Child Development, 67,* 91–103.

Ogunniyi, A., Lekwauwa, U. G., & Osuntokun, B. O. (1991). Influence of education on aspects of cognitive functions in non-demented elderly Nigerians. *Neuroepidemiology, 10,* 246–250.

Ogunniyi, A., & Osuntokun, B. (1991). Relatively low prevalence of Alzheimer's disease in developing countries, and the racial factor in dementia research. *Ethnicity and Disease, 1,* 394–395.

Osuntokun, B. O., Ogunniyi, A. O., Lekwauwa, U. G., Norton, Jr., J. A., & Pillay, N. (1992). Cross-cultural studies in Alzheimer's disease. *Ethnicity and Disease, 2,* 352–357.

Owan, T. C., Bliatout, B., Lin, K-M., Liu, W., Nguyen, T. D., & Wong, H. Z. (Eds.). (1985). *Southeast*

Asian mental health: Treatment, prevention, training, and research (DHHS Publication No. ADM 85-1399). Washington, DC: U.S. Government Printing Office.

Pang, V. O. (1988). Ethnic prejudice: Still alive and hurtful. *Harvard Educational Review, 58,* 375–379.

Pang, V. O., & Barba, R. (1995). The power of culture: Building culturally affirming instruction. In C. Grant (Ed.), *Educating for diversity* (pp. 341–358). Needham Heights, MA: Allyn & Bacon.

Pang, V. O., Gay, G., & Stanley, W. B. (1995). Expanding conceptions of community and civic competence for a multicultural society. *Theory and Research in Social Education, 23,* 302–331.

Paniagua, F. A. (1994). *Assessing and treating culturally diverse clients: A practical guide.* Thousand Oaks, CA: Sage.

Patterson, M. B., & Bolger, J. P. (1994). Assessment of behavioral symptoms in Alzheimer disease. *Alzheimer Disease and Associated Disorders, 8*(Suppl. 3), 3–20.

Pedraza, S., & Rumbaut, R. G. (1996). *Origins and destinies: Immigration, race, and ethnicity in America.* Belmont, CA: Wadsworth.

Phanthumchinda, K., Jitapunkul, S., Sitthi-Amorn, C., & Bunnag, S. C. (1991). Prevalence of dementia in an urban slum population in Thailand: Validity of screening methods. *International Journal of Geriatric Psychiatry, 6,* 639–646.

Phillipson, M., Moranville, J. T., Jeste, D. V., & Harris, J. M. (1990). Antipsychotics. *Clinics in Geriatric Medicine, 6,* 411–422.

Pi, J., Olive, P. M., Roca, J., & Masana, L. (1996). Prevalence of dementia in a semi-rural population of Catalunya, Spain. *Neuroepidemiology, 15,* 33–41.

Pickett, M. (1993). Cultural awareness in the context of terminal illness. *Cancer Nursing, 16*(2), 102–106.

Popenoe, D. (1971). *Sociology.* New York: Meredith.

Poplin, M., & Phillips, L. (1993). Sociocultural aspects of language and literacy: Issues facing educators of students with learning disabilities. *Learning Disability Quarterly, 16,* 245–255.

Powell, L. S., & Courtice, K. (1990). *Enfermedad de Alzheimer: Una guia para la familia* [Alzheimer's disease: A guide for families]. México, D.F.: Editorial Pax México.

Purdy, J. K., & Arguello, D. (1992). Hispanic familism in caretaking of older adults: Is it functional? *Journal of Gerontological Social Work, 19,* 29–43.

Queralt, M. (1996). *The social environment and human behavior: A diversity perspective.* Needham Heights, MA: Allyn & Bacon.

Ridley, C. R., & Lingle, D. W. (1996). Cultural empathy in multicultural counseling. In P. B. Pedersen, J. G. Draguns, W. L. Lonner, & J. E. Trimble (Eds.), Counseling across cultures (pp. 21–46). Thousand Oaks, CA: Sage Publications.

Rivera, F. G., & Erlich, J. L. (1992). *Community organizing in a diverse society.* Needham Heights, MA: Allyn & Bacon.

Rogers, M. F. (1996). *Multicultural experiences, multicultural theories.* New York: McGraw-Hill.

Rogler, L. H. (1993). Culture in psychiatric diagnosis: An issue of scientific accuracy. *Psychiatry, 56,* 324–327.

Rogler, L. H., & Cortes, D. E. (1993). Help-seeking pathways: A unifying concept in mental health care. *American Journal of Psychiatry, 150,* 554–561.

Ross, G. W., Abbott, R. D., Petrovich, H., Masaki, K. H., Murdaugh, C., Trockerman, C., Curb, J. D., & White, L. R. (1997). Frequency and characteristics of silent dementia among elderly Japanese-American men. *Journal of the American Medical Association, 277*(10), 800–805.

Rossenthal, C. (1986). Family support in later life: Does ethnicity makes a difference? *The Gerontologist, 26,* 19–24.

Sachs, G. A., & Cassell, C. K. (1989). Ethical aspects of dementia. *Neurologic Clinics, 7,* 846–859.

Sakauye, K. M., Baker, F. M., Chacko, R. C., Jimenez, R. G., Nickens, H. W., & Thompson, J. W. (Eds.). (1994). *Ethnic minority elderly: A task force report of the American Psychiatric Association.* Washington, DC: American Psychiatric Association.

Saldov, M., & Chow, P. (1994). The ethnic elderly in metro Toronto hospitals, nursing homes, and homes for the aged: Communication and health care. *International Journal of Aging and Human Development, 38,* 117–135.

Samovar, L. A., & Porter, R. E. (1995). *Communication between cultures* (2nd ed.). Belmont, CA: Wadsworth.

Saunders, A. M., Strittmatter, W. J., Schmechel, D., St. George-Hyslop, P. H., Pericak-Vance, M. A., Joo, S. H., Rosi, B. L., Gusella, J. F., Crapper-MacLachlan, D. R., Alberts, M. J., Hulette, C., Crain, G., Goldgaber, D., & Roses, A. D. (1993). Association of apolipoprotein E allele e4 with late-onset and sporadic Alzheimer's disease. *Neurology, 43,* 1467–1472.

Schatzman, L., & Strauss, A. L. (1973). *Field research: Strategies for a natural sociology.* Englewood Cliffs, NJ: Prentice Hall.

Schneider-Corey, M., & Corey, G. (1992). *Groups: Process and practice* (4th ed.). Pacific Grove, CA: Brooks/Cole.

Schoenberg, B. S., Anderson, D. W., & Haerer, A. F. (1985). Severe dementia: Prevalence and clinical features in a biracial U.S. population. *Archives of Neurology, 42,* 740–743.

Schrafft, G. (1980). Nursing home care and the minority elderly. *Journal of Long Term Care Administration, 8,* 1–31.

Segal, M., & Wykle, M. (1988–1989). The black family's experience with dementia. *Journal of Applied Social Sciences, 13,* 170–191.

Serby, M., Chou, J. C-Y., & Franssen, E. H. (1987). Dementia in an American-Chinese nursing home population. *American Journal of Psychiatry, 144,* 811–812.

Siddarthan, K., & Sowers-Hoag, K. (1989). Elders' attitudes and access to health care: A comparison of Cuban immigrants and native-born Americans. *Journal of Applied Gerontology, 8,* 86–96.

Silva-Netto, B. R. (1994). Cultural symbols and images in the counseling process. *Pastoral Psychology, 42,* 277–284.

Sirkin, M. I. (1994, July/August). Resisting cultural meltdown. *Networker,* pp. 48–52.

Sizemore, M. T., Ochoa-Coover, M., West, H. L., & Mahon, J. (1991). Translating Alzheimer's disease education videotapes into Spanish. *Journal of Biocommunication, 18,* 2–6.

Smart, J. F., & Smart, D. W. (1993). Acculturation, biculturalism, and the rehabilitation of Mexican Americans. *Journal of Applied Rehabilitation Counseling, 24*(3), 46–51.

Smith, S. A. (1975). *Natural systems and the elderly: An unrecognized resource.* Portland, OR: Portland State University School of Social Work.

Smyth, K., Whitehouse, P. J., Rust, M., & Khaana, J. (1988–1989). Epidemiology, diagnosis, and management of Alzheimer's disease and related disorders: Implications for minority populations. *Health Matrix, 6,* 28–33.

Sokolovsky, J. (1990). Bringing culture back home: Aging, ethnicity, and family support. In J. Sokolovsky (Ed.), *The cultural context of aging: Worldwide perspectives* (pp. 201–211). New York: Bergin & Garvey.

Song, Y. I., & Kim, E. C. (1993). *American mosaic: Selected readings on America's multicultural heritage.* Englewood Cliffs, NJ: Prentice Hall.

Sotomayor, M., & Curriel, H. (1988). *Hispanic elderly: A cultural signature.* Edinburgh, TX: Pan American University Press.

Sreenivasan, S. (1996, July 22). As mainstream papers struggle, the ethnic press is thriving. *New York Times,* p. C7.

Stanford, E. P., & Torres-Gil, F. M. (1991). Diversity and beyond: A commentary. *Generations, 15,* 5–7.

Stein, H. F. (1990). *American medicine as culture.* Boulder, CO: Westview Press.

Stern, Y., Andrews, H., Puttman, J., Sano, M., Tatemichi, T., Lantigua, R., & Mayeux, R. (1992). Diagnosis in dementia in a heterogeneous population: Development of a neuropsychological paradigm-based diagnosis of dementia and quantified correction for the effects of education. *Archives of Neurology, 49,* 453–460.

Stewart, E. C. (1972). *American cultural patterns: A cross-cultural perspective.* LaGrange Park, IL: Intercultural Network.

Strickland, T. L., Ranganath, V., Lin, K-M., Poland, R. E., Mendoza, R., & Smith, M. W. (1991). Psychopharmacologic considerations in the treatment of black American populations. *Psychopharmacology Bulletin, 27,* 441–448.

Strong, C. (1984). Stress and caring for elderly relatives: Interpretations and coping strategies in an American Indian and white sample. *The Gerontologist, 24,* 251–256.

Sue, D. W., & Sue, D. (1990). *Counseling the culturally different.* New York: Wiley.

Suttles, G. D. (1972). *The social construction of communities.* Chicago: University of Chicago Press.

Szapocznik, J., & Kurtines, W. M. (1993). Family psychology and cultural diversity: Opportunities for theory, research, and application. *American Psychologist, 48,* 400–407.

Talamantes, M. A., Cornell, J., Espino, D.V., Lichtenstein, M. J., & Hazuda, H. P. (1996). SES and ethnic differences in perceived caregiver availability among young-old Mexican Americans and non-Hispanic whites. *The Gerontologist, 36,* 88–99.

Tallmer, M., Mayer, M., & Hill, G. (1977). Cross-cultural issues in nursing home settings. *Journal of Geriatric Psychiatry, 10,* 173–189.

Taussig, I. M., Henderson, V. W., & Mack, W. (1992). Spanish translation and validation of a neuropsychological battery: Performance of Spanish- and English-speaking Alzheimer's disease patients and normal comparison subjects. *Clinical Gerontologist, 11,* 95–108.

Taussig, M. I., & Trejo, L. (1992). Outreach to Spanish-speaking caregivers of persons with memory impairments: A brief report. *Clinical Gerontologist, 13,* 183–195.

Taylor, O. L. (1992). The effects of cultural assumptions on cross-cultural communication. In D. R. Koslow & E. P. Salett (Eds.), *Crossing cultures in mental health* (pp. 18–27). Washington, DC: SIETAR International.

Taylor, R. J., Neighbors, H. W., & Broman, C. L. (1989). Evaluation by black Americans of a social service encounter during a serious personal problem. *Social Work, 34,* 193–288.

Tempo, P. M., & Saito, A. (1996). Techniques of working with Japanese American families. In G. Yeo & D. Gallagher-Thompson (Eds.), *Ethnicity and the dementias* (pp. 109–122). Washington, DC: Taylor and Francis.

Ten warning signs of Alzheimer's disease, the. (1995). Chicago, IL: Alzheimer's Association.

Teri, L., & Gallagher-Thompson, D. (1991). Cognitive–behavioral interventions for treatment of depression in Alzheimer's patients. *The Gerontologist, 31,* 413–416.

Teri, L., Rabins, P., Whitehouse, P., Berg, L., Reisberg, B., Sunderland, T., Eichelman, B., & Crighton, P. (1992). Management of behavior disturbance in Alzheimer disease: Current knowledge and future directions. *Alzheimer Disease and Associated Disorders, 6,* 77–88.

Thiederman, S. (1991). *Bridging cultural barriers for corporate success: How to manage the multicultural workforce.* New York: Lexington Books.

Thomas, Jr., R. R. (1994). From affirmative action to affirming diversity. In M. C. Gentile (Ed.), *Differences that work: Organizational excellence through diversity* (pp. 27–46). Boston: Harvard Business Review Book Series.

Thomas, V. J., & Rose, F. D. (1991). Ethnic differences in the experience of pain. *Social Science and Medicine, 32,* 1063–1066.

Tombaugh, T. N., & McIntyre, N. J. (1992). The Mini-Mental State Examination: A comprehensive review. *Journal of the American Geriatric Society, 40,* 922–935.

Torres Gil, F., & Fiedler, E. (1986–1987). Long term care policy and the Hispanic population. *Journal of Hispanic Policy, 2,* 49–66.

Triandis, H. (1978). Approaches toward minimizing translation. In R. Brislin (Ed.), *Translation: Applications and research* (pp. 229–243). New York. Wiley/Halstead.

Triandis, H. C., Bontempo, R., Leung, K., & Hui, C. H. (1990). A method for determining cultural, demographic, and personal constructs. *Journal of Cross-Cultural Psychology, 21,* 302–318.

Triandis, H. C., Kurowski, L., Tecktiel, A., & Chan, D. (1993). Extracting the emics of diversity. *International Journal of Intercultural Relations, 17,* 217–234.

Trimble, J. E., Fleming, C. M., Beauvis, F., & Jumper-Thrurman, P. (1996). Essential cultural and social strategies for counseling Native American Indians. In P. B. Pedersen, J. G. Draguns, W. L. Lonner, & J. F. Trimble (Eds.), *Counseling across cultures* (pp. 177–209). Thousand Oaks, CA: Sage Publications.

Tropman, J. E., Erlich, J. L., & Rothman, J. (Eds.). (1995). *Tactics and techniques of community intervention.* Itaska, IL: F. E. Peacock.

Tune, L. E., Steele, C., & Cooper, T. (1991). Neuroleptic drugs in the management of behavioral symptoms of Alzheimer's disease. *Psychiatric Clinics of North America, 14,* 353–373.

U.S. Congress Office of Technology Assessment. (1987). *Losing a million minds: Confronting the tragedy of Alzheimer's disease and other dementias* (Publication No. OTA-BA-323). Washington, DC: U.S. Government Printing Office.

U.S. Congress Office of Technology Assessment. (1990). *Confused minds, burdened families: Finding help for people with Alzheimer's disease and other dementias* (Publication No. OTA-BA-403). Washington, DC: U.S. Government Printing Office.

U.S. Department of Education. (1993). *Adult literacy in America.* Washington, DC: National Center for Education Statistics, U.S. Department of Education.

Valle, R. (1980a). A natural resource system for health–mental health promotion to Latino/Hispanic populations. In R. Valle & W. Vega (Eds.), *Hispanic natural support systems: Mental health promotion perspectives* (pp. 35–43). Sacramento: State of California Department of Mental Health.

Valle, R. (1980b). Social mapping techniques: A preliminary guide for locating and linking to natural networks. In R. Valle & W. Vega (Eds.), *Hispanic natural support systems: Mental health promotion perspectives* (pp. 113–121). Sacramento: State of California Department of Mental Health.

Valle, R. (1981). Natural support systems, minority groups, and the late life dementias: Implications for service delivery, research and policy. In N. E. Miller & G. D. Cohen (Eds.), *Clinical aspects of Alzheimer's disease and senile dementia* (Vol. 15, pp. 277–299). New York: Raven Press.

Valle, R. (1985). Hispanic social networks and prevention. In R. Hough, P. A. Gongola, V. B. Brown, & S. E. Goldston (Eds.), *Psychiatric epidemiology and prevention: The possibilities* (pp. 131–157). Los Angeles: University of California at Los Angeles, Neuropsychatric Institute.

Valle, R. (1988–1989). Outreach to ethnic minorities with Alzheimer's disease: The challenge to the community. *Health Matrix, 6,* 13–27.

Valle, R. (1989). U.S. ethnic minority group access to long-term care. In T. Schwab (Ed.), *Caring for an aging world: International models for long-term care, financing, and delivery* (pp. 339–365). New York: McGraw-Hill.

Valle, R. (1990a). Cultural and ethnic issues in Alzheimer's disease family research. In E. Light & B. D. Lebowitz (Eds.), *Alzheimer's disease treatment and family stress: Directions for research* (pp. 122–154). Washington, DC: Taylor and Francis.

Valle, R. (1990b). The Latino/Hispanic family and their elderly: Approaches to cross-cultural curriculum design in the health professions. In M. S. Harper (Ed.), *Minority aging: Essential curricula content for selected health and allied professions* (pp. 433–452; DHHS Publication No. HRS PDV-904). Washington, DC: U.S. Government Printing Office.

Valle, R. (1992a). A Hispanic initiative in Alzheimer's disease and related disorders research. In *Hispanic aging, Parts I & II* (pp. 106–122). Washington, DC: National Institute on Aging.

Valle, R. (1992b). Providing long term care services to ethnic minority elders with dementing diseases. In J. E. Jackson, R. Katzman, & P. J. Lessin (Eds.), *Alzheimer's disease: Long term care* (pp. 153–158). San Diego, CA: San Diego University Press.

Valle, R. (1994). Culture-fair behavioral symptom differential assessment and intervention in dementing illness. *Alzheimer Disease and Associated Disorders, 8*(Suppl. 3), 21–45.

Valle, R., & Bensussen, G. (1986). Hispanic social networks, social support, and mental health. In W. M. Vega & M. R. Miranda (Eds.), *Stress and Hispanic mental health. Relating research to service delivery* (pp. 147–173; DHHS Publication No. ADM 85-1410). Washington, DC: U.S. Government Printing Office.

Valle, R., Birba, L., Yelder, J., Sakamoto-Kowalchuck, Y., Forquera, R., Cosgrove, R., & Neleson, D. (1989). *Linking ethnic minority elderly with dementia to long term care services* (U.S. Congress Office of Technology Assessment Contract Report No. H-36640-0). Springfield, VA: National Technical Information Service.

Valle, R., & Martinez, C. (1985). Natural networks of elderly Latinos of Mexican heritage: Implications for mental health. In M. Miranda & R. A. Ruiz (Eds.), *Chicano aging and mental health* (pp. 76–117; DHHS Publication No. ADM 81-952). Washington, DC: U.S. Government Printing Office.

Valle, R., & Mendoza, L. (1978). *The Latino elder.* San Diego, CA: Campanile Press.

Valle, R., Willis, L., Vega, S., & Cook Gait, E. (1994). La evaluación neuropsicolgica y transcultural de la demencia senil: La experiencia entre el grupo Latino, Norteamericano [Conducting a transcultural neuropsychological evaluation of dementing illness in a North American Latino population]. In J. Buendia (Ed.), *Envejecimiento y psicología de la salud* (pp. 313–339). Madrid, Spain: Editores, S.A.

van der Cammen, T. J. M., & van Harskamp, F. (1992). Value of the Mini-Mental State Examination in an informants' data for the detection of dementia in geriatric outpatients. *Psychological Reports, 71,* 1003–1009.

Vega, W. A., & Murphy, J. W. (1990). *Culture and the restructuring of community mental health.* New York: Greenwood Press.

Vidich, A. J., Bensman, J., & Stein, M. R. (1964). *Reflections on community studies.* New York: Wiley.

Wallace, S. P. (1990). The no-care zone: Availability, accessibility, and acceptability in community-based long term care. *The Gerontologist, 30,* 254–261.

Wallace, S. P., Campbell, K., & Lew-Ting, C-Y. (1994). Structural barriers to the use of formal in-home services by elderly Latinos. *Journal of Gerontology: Social Sciences, 49,* S353–S263.

Warren, R. L. (1955). *Studying your community.* New York: Free Press.

Warren, R. L. (1973). *The community in America.* New York: Rand McNally.

Welsh, K. A., Ballad, E., Nash, F., Raiford, K., & Harrel, L. (1994). Issues affecting minority participation in research studies of Alzheimer's disease. *Alzheimer Disease and Associated Disorders, 8* (Suppl. 4), 38–48.

Wershow, H. J. (1976). Inadequate census data on black nursing home patients. *The Gerontologist, 16,* 86–87.

Westermeyer, J. (1987). Cultural factors in clinical assessment. *Journal of Consulting and Clinical Psychology, 55,* 471–478.

Wood, J. B., & Parham, I. A. (1990). Coping with perceived burden: Ethnic and cultural issues in Alzheimer's family caregiving. *Journal of Applied Gerontology, 9,* 325–339.

Wykle, M., & Segal, M. (1991). A comparison of black and white family caregivers with dementia. *Journal of the National Black Nurses Association, 5,* 28–41.

Yancy Martin, P., & O'Connor, G. G. (1989). *The social environment: Open systems applications.* New York: Longman.

Yaniz, M. J. (1990). *Geriatric assessment: Risks of functional disability, dementia, and depression, among Hispanic elderly living at home with caregivers' support.* Unpublished doctoral dissertation, Illinois Institute of Technology, Chicago.

Yeo, G., Gallagher-Thompson, D., & Lieberman, M. (1996). Variations in dementia characteristics by ethnic category. In G. Yeo & D. Gallagher-Thompson (Eds.), *Ethnicity and the dementias* (pp. 21–30). Washington, DC: Taylor and Francis.

Young, R. F., & Kahana, E. (1995). The context of caregiving and well-being outcomes among African and Caucasian Americans. *The Gerontologist, 35,* 225–232.

Young, R. F., Solakumni, E., Young, J. H., & Peters, J. (1996). Issues of recruitment and retention in Alzheimer's research among African and White Americans. *Journal of Aging and Ethnicity, 1,* 19–25.

Yu, E. S. H., Liu, W. T., Levy, P., Zhang, M-Y., Katzman, R., Lung, C-T., Wong, S-C., Wang, Z-Y., & Qu, G-Y. (1989). Cognitive impairment among elderly adults in Shanghai, China. *Journal of Gerontology: Social Sciences, 44,* S97–106.

Zastrow, C. (1985). *Social work with groups.* Chicago: Nelson-Hall.

Zhang, Z-X., Anderson, D. W., Lavine, L., & Mantel, N. (1990). Geographic patterns of Parkinson–dementia complex on Guam. *Archives of Neurology, 47,* 1069–1074.

Index